Food Allergy Survivors Together Handbook

Food Allergy Survivors Together Handbook

By Melissa Taylor

Writers Club Press
San Jose New York Lincoln Shanghai

Food Allergy Survivors Together Handbook

All Rights Reserved © 2002 by Melissa Taylor

No part of this book may be reproduced or transmitted in any form or by any means, graphic, electronic, or mechanical, including photocopying, recording, taping, or by any information storage retrieval system, without the permission in writing from the publisher.

Writers Club Press
an imprint of iUniverse, Inc.

For information address:
iUniverse, Inc.
5220 S. 16th St., Suite 200
Lincoln, NE 68512
www.iuniverse.com

Nothing in this book should be construed as medical advice. People with food allergies should be under the care of an allergist and direct medical questions toward him or her.

ISBN: 0-595-24128-X

Printed in the United States of America

Contents

Introduction ix

Chapter 1	My Story 1
Chapter 2	Dealing with Others 9
Chapter 3	Strange Reactions 23
Chapter 4	Making Food Fun Again 27
Chapter 5	Allergists, Doctors, and Medications 33
Chapter 6	Eating Out 41
Chapter 7	Finding Something to Do 47
Chapter 8	Less Common Allergies 57
Chapter 9	Shopping 61
Chapter 10	Reading and Understanding Labels 67
Chapter 11	Allergens in Non-Food Items 75
Chapter 12	When Doubt Sets In 77
Chapter 13	The Little Things 81
Chapter 14	Where Are the Recipes? 83
Chapter 15	Your Experience Can Change Lives 87
Chapter 16	Christmas and Other Holidays 91
Chapter 17	Traveling 97
Chapter 18	I'm All Alone 101

Chapter 19	Further Resources	107
Chapter 20	A Chapter for Those Who Don't Have Allergies	111
Conclusion		115
Appendix	"My Tips for Someone Newly Diagnosed"	117
About the Author		121

Acknowledgements

I can't in good conscience present this book without giving thanks to the people who provided me with ideas and financial support in its writing and publication.

To FAST visitors: I am grateful for your input toward making this a useful handbook for people with food allergies. All of your ideas and suggestions made me aware of topics that people with food allergies are concerned about. If I listed specific names, I know I would leave someone out, so I will just say "thank you" to everyone!

To my parents: Thank you for believing in this book enough to help with the finances required to make it available to the public. Thank you also for supporting me during my years of learning to live with food allergies.

Introduction

When I was diagnosed with food allergies at sixteen years of age, my immediate questions were not medical in nature. Instead of asking myself where I got them, what they were caused by, or how a test for food allergies works, I was mostly concerned with how my life would change. Food is important to anyone, but especially to the American teenager. The diagnosis was, of course, a relief in a way. After all, I knew the source of sixteen years of unexplained symptoms and illnesses. More on my mind, though, was that my life as I knew it had reached a close. I would need to start eating differently, thinking differently. In a way, I was an entirely different person.

I was suddenly a person with a label. I was a disabled person who needed to watch her diet carefully, who would potentially never graduate from high school due to excessive absences. I longed for someone to talk to. For someone to say, "I know what you have been through. Sit down and we'll talk."

My purpose in writing this book is to be that person for you. This book is meant to be upbeat and funny. It's intended to be something you will pick up when you need to hear from someone who understands, when you need a bit of encouragement, or simply need an idea of something to do that doesn't involve eating.

In a survey conducted on the FAST website with 800 participants, which asked what age group was afflicted with food allergies, 50% of those with the condition reported to be age 17 or older. However, the resources available for people with food allergies are generally geared toward parents (usually mothers) of children with food allergies. Due to the lack of attention from the media, we often feel alienated and alone with our circumstances.

Though this book is intended for adults with food allergies, it is also my hope that parents of children with food allergies will find useful information within its pages.

Regardless of your situation—whether a teen with food allergies, an adult with food allergies, or a parent of an allergic child—it is my wish that you will find that a diagnosis does not necessarily need to be taken as negative. Though your life will be different, others have been there, too, and working together can make life with allergies more manageable. That knowledge in itself is the mission of Food Allergy Survivors Together.

Melissa Taylor
Founder of FAST
www.angelfire.com/mi/FAST

P.S. Nothing in this book should be construed as medical advice or medical information. Everything within these pages is merely based on the opinion and experience of the author. If you have any questions, please consult your allergist.

1

My Story

A Difficult Start

As a newborn I could have owned the patent on crying, and a quarter of a century later my parents still talk about it, so it must have been quite impressive. Despite a large unexplained rash and visits to the pediatrician, however, he told them that there was nothing wrong with me (other than being a cry-baby).

As the years passed there were other symptoms that came along. Black circles under my eyes, severe stomachaches, diarrhea, and vomiting became more and more common. Because doctors were always unable to explain away the symptoms, it became more and more common to believe that I had emotional, rather than physical, problems. My "frail nature" apparently made me more prone to getting sick, and also to developing frequent ailments such as ear and sinus infections and bronchitis.

My teachers were just as confused as my parents. One teacher noticed my brother, eighteen months older, at school and asked him why I was absent so much. "She has bad emotional problems," was my brother's reply.

My parents were at a loss. They didn't know what to do with me. To give them credit, doctors were just as much to blame, because they were unable to find the root cause of my strange health problems. If I vomited and had diarrhea and a temperature of 96.0, they would give me the diagnosis of having a bad case of the intestinal flu. With the scaly, open, oozing sores behind my ears (now we know that this is called "eczema"), my mom would tell me it was because I didn't wash behind my ears enough.

I knew that even though I was in physical pain every day of my life, there was no way for anyone to believe me because doctors didn't even have an answer. When I was about fifteen years old I was misdiagnosed with a condition called an "acidic stomach." Despite the fact that the prescribed medication never helped, I tried to hang on to that diagnosis, because it was the first time in fifteen years that I had something to blame rather than my emotional state. For once I could tell people that I really had something wrong with me.

Could all of my health problems possibly have been in my head? After all, the medication wasn't helping. In a journal, dated September of 1993, I wrote, "This is so stupid! I am tired of going to the doctor, tired of being sick, tired of missing school, tired of doing makeup homework, tired of being home, tired of being cooped up inside, tired of getting made fun of because I am sick."

Though at first I wasn't sick enough for doctors to really notice a trend, my illnesses and minor complaints gradually increased in frequency and severity. My journal shows the gradual progression of my questioning the legitimacy of my illnesses toward finally accepting that I was genuinely ill, even if I didn't know why I had so many strange symptoms. Previously, my family and I just believed I was "delicate." One time an attack of throwing up accompanied with diarrhea was attributed to working too hard on a craft. Another time it was credited to writing too much in my journal. After a while, however, it became very obvious that there was something seriously wrong with me.

In early 1994 it was decided that I would be tested for allergies…as in seasonal and inhalant allergies. (My parents believed that my pets might be responsible for my health problems.) The allergist gave me 50 pricks in my back and tested me for inhalant and seasonal allergies. No welts formed. I was, actually, quite relieved. I've always been an animal fan, because during my times of losing friends and people questioning my sanity, they were some of the only comrades and confidants I had.

The last thing I wanted was to be allergic to animals. Then, because those tests were all negative, I had "the third blood-letting I've had" (according to my journal) in less than four months. I was beginning to feel like a human pincushion after being tested for so many illnesses, but it led me to develop my own philosophy with needles. Keep your eye on the second-hand of the room wall clock, and you'll do fine! Anyway, from my symptoms and family history of allergies, the MD allergist was somewhat sure that I had food allergies. However, after years of negative tests I basically believed these would also come back negative, and in my journal I only referred to them in a casual manner. In fact, according to my journal, even while the test was being sent off my mom was convinced that I instead had anemia. To further show my skepticism of any allergies to food, the journal ends before the test results even came back!

As you probably already knew before you decided to read this book (the title is somewhat a giveaway, I suppose!), the tests came back positive. Very positive. My milk allergy was completely off the chart, and wheat was almost too high to register, as well. My main allergies are wheat, all gluten-containing grains, dairy, soy, peanuts, and eggs.

FASTing

What often surprises people about the founding of FAST (which is now an Internet support group and website for people with allergies in the family) is that it was a teenager who founded it.

My immediate reaction after learning that I had "moderately severe" multiple food allergies (to quote the allergist) was to yearn to find out more about them from others who were "in the know." I knew nothing, nada, zip. The whole idea of being allergic to foods—actually getting sick from eating (which was as normal as breathing)—sounded crazy, although I believed the test results and the doctor's diagnosis.

It wasn't long before I came up with the idea of a free computer-printed newsletter to distribute in our local health food store. The entire goal would be for me to find other people in our town with food allergies, and to swap recipes, tips, and emotional support through this means. My mom, brother and I were headed somewhere in our van when I told them about my desire to write a newsletter. This may come as a shock to some. Where did a sixteen year old come up with the idea of a newsletter? But it wasn't all that unusual. Ever since I was about eleven years old I had been writing and editing a newsletter for my pen pals. I loved to write and speak out on my opinions. So it was only natural for me to suggest a newsletter.

My mom, brother and I all agreed that it was an interesting idea, and worth pursuing. So, still in the van, my mom promised to speak to the health food store's owners to see if they would be willing to hand out the newsletter, and then we all happily brain-stormed for a name. My brother came up with the acronym "FAST," which he intended to be tongue-in-cheek. Many people think "fast" means "quick," or that it's simply a meaningless acronym, but this is not so. It means "fasting," which is the cutting out of certain foods—sometimes all foods—in one's diet. I didn't understand this, but my brother and mom laughed over the double meaning of the name. I don't think it was until a few years later that I actually understood his joke!

To spell out the entire acronym, he came up with the name "Food Allergy Sufferers Together." My mom balked at that idea. "Sufferers" sounded really negative. "How about 'survivors' instead?" And that's how the name was born.

The newsletter's original intention was to help us as well as to offer help to others. Financially it was a bit of a problem, since we offered it for free. Coming up with new ideas was draining me, especially since only one person contacted us with input (a recipe, and it used spelt (which is basically wheat, which I had been advised to avoid)). We stopped with the newsletter after what I believe was about a year.

In 1997 I came home from my early morning classes at my first semester of college and logged into our newly acquired Internet connection. I decided to surf for food allergy information, but was surprised to find out there was, I believe, only one site about food allergies (would you believe that now? Probably not). Already knowing a bit of HTML (a website programming language) from having done personal pages for fun, I set up a site with recipes, book reviews, and cooking tips. The site was completely intended for adults with food allergies.

After submitting it to search engines I waited for people to come, and was surprised at FAST's very speedy popularity. It became evident that other people had also desired a way to speak with others who have food allergies. Since we may not know of others with food allergies in our hometowns, since it is not a very common disorder, the Internet is an incredibly practical means of communicating with them.

My original vision for FAST was to be a place for adults with allergies to network. However, parents of children with food allergies also needed a place to "meet" and share ideas. Therefore, the vision of the Internet FAST from very early on has been for all ages to be welcomed and embraced.

School

When I hear that people are having problems with their children who have food allergies in regards to schooling—on occasion such serious problems that some of them end up having to home-school their children—I am saddened, but I also understand. I know just how hard it is and how frustrating it is to have difficulties when dealing with a school.

Before we found out about my allergies I went to public school. They had a strict attendance policy. If I missed more days than the school allowed I had to obtain doctor permits to prove I was legitimately sick. Unfortunately, the doctors treated the symptoms and not the underlying problem. Some teachers seemed to be skeptical of my unexplained, frequent, and undiagnosed illnesses.

When I was finally diagnosed at age sixteen the allergist wrote a quick note to my school explaining that my lifelong problems were due to severe food allergies, and that they should help me with special needs I might have. The school began by hiring a tutor (an employee of the public school system and not an actual tutor or teacher) to teach me at home. Unfortunately, she did very unprofessional things, such as calling up last-minute to say she would come after dinner, or she would simply not show up at all (on more than one occasion). She even asked me to drop a class since she didn't like it. A journal entry from March 15, 1994 explains my confusion and frustration with the tutor: "She said she 'totally forgot,' but I don't believe it. She's been late four times [and has] only showed up three times so far." The school changed to a real tutor when they realized she was skipping our meetings, which was really stressing me out further in my already beleaguered state. The real tutor was a substitute teacher who was exceptionally nice and very helpful. Unfortunately, they didn't switch to her until close to the end of the school year. Because of their lack of preparation for a person with special needs I didn't take enough credits to "pass" my junior year.

During my second attempt at a junior year I was well enough to attend school on a regular basis. They cut down my class load to four credits, and I went home in the afternoons before lunchtime.

In my senior year of high school I became very ill again. Generally these bouts of extreme, long illnesses were due to ingesting allergens I didn't know about. For example, I was ingesting milk products, when I'm in fact allergic to them. (I didn't understand labeling at that time.)

I decided to make the very disappointing decision to drop out in around October of my senior year. To be so close to graduating and to give up on it was incredibly discouraging. My life seemed to be headed nowhere.

For a while, I was the stereotypical high school dropout, staying at home sleeping away the days. Of course, my reasons were a bit better than the reasons of most dropouts! My mom had in the back of her mind the memory that someone she used to work with had had a daughter in an at-home school program. After my mom got in contact with her I applied to enter the program and was accepted. I got a legitimate high-school degree from a high school in the United States (rather than a G.E.D.). I had a different teacher for each subject, an advisor, etc. I ended up graduating from a high school that I will forever have good, instead of bad memories about…especially because it was my favorite year of school! What first looked like a terrible senior year ended up being a delightful experience! I will admit that I missed out on social aspects of having a senior year in a public high school, but my friends had already graduated and moved on by that time (since I was a year behind), so it did not seem like a big loss.

Getting into college was another problem. I had to talk to someone there about my situation, and I felt (perhaps wrongly so) as if he really talked down to me. Instead of addressing my health concerns, he made it appear that he was concerned about my grades. Although I didn't understand this at the time, I now believe that this is because schools are not allowed to prohibit you from coming due to health problems, but are allowed to discriminate against people with poor grades. I believe he said I needed to have a C-average for my senior year to get in (I got a 4.0 (straight As)). I left confused and sad. However, I did end up getting accepted.

I only take a few credits each semester at the college, in order to not over-tax myself. Sometimes I've had to take a half or even a full semester off to get back to where I feel well enough to attend.

I feel that no matter what grade you are in—from grade school on up—you will face prejudice (or innocent misunderstandings) due to your health problems. I had one college teacher who refused to be lenient on my grade because I had missed one or two extra days than she allowed (she put everyone down 1/2 grade per "extra" absence). Despite having a legitimate disability we must realize that throughout our lives not everyone is going to accept it as an excuse for being absent, or for being incapable of certain things, even though I would assume that most teachers would prefer I be absent than vomiting or fainting in school (I've done both!).

I also need to remember to be tolerant, because food allergies are not a highly understood disease. Many people think of food allergies as something that gives you slight sniffles or asthma, or they believe food allergies are like lactose intolerance. I need to stop being upset with people, and instead use these types of experiences as opportunities to educate them about my problem.

2

Dealing with Others

The misunderstandings I have had with schools and teachers lead, of course, to the topic of dealing with people in general.

There is one primary rule to keep in mind. That is this: *I must realize people don't know what food allergies are.*

This sounds like an incredibly bold statement to make. "People don't know what food allergies are?!" But think about it. Before you were diagnosed, how many times did you think about food allergies? How often did you research them? How much did you know? Hindsight is 20/20. When I was little my brother's friend had food allergies. I just thought it was sort of strange. I believed he really had them, but I had no interest in learning more about food allergies in general, or what they did to him. Like most people, I perceived food as harmless; something that is basic and essential for everyday life. The fact that food can be dangerous to certain people is a hard fact to grasp. Because of this, it can seem as though people are exaggerating or making up their illness.

Most people probably don't really want to know more.

As someone who has food allergies, sometimes I feel like I want to educate the world. However, the world doesn't necessarily want to be educated. How many times have you found out that someone has a disease, only to want to learn everything you could about it? Most likely, this has never happened. If you *have* researched a friend or acquaintance's disorder, then you should give yourself a pat on the back. For the most part people aren't going to make the effort to fully understand your condition. You can't really expect them to.

Because I tended to hide my symptoms over the years, and because my friends believed they were due to certain temporary illnesses (such as the flu and colds), I had a hard time convincing them about my allergies. My best friend growing up, while talking to me long-distance, admitted that she didn't remember me frequently being sick or being absent from school. A past good friend, whom I knew at a later age, ran into me and started talking about my acidic stomach. I had to remind her that *that* diagnosis was a *mis*diagnosis, and that I really have food allergies. My friends today are also confused with anything and everything having to do with food allergies. One friend was convinced at one time that people get them due to not exercising.

Many don't realize that food allergies can be serious and even life threatening. They don't realize that labels on foods are not completely comprehensive and do not necessarily list all of their ingredients. They don't understand that eating out in a restaurant is potentially a threat to our health and perhaps even to our lives.

You have probably seen the type of ribbing that people who are on a voluntary diet for weight-loss reasons encounter. "Try it. A little won't hurt," their friends taunt them over desserts. Individuals with food allergies may be treated this way as well…but the problem is that, with us, it can and it *will* hurt.

We seem to worship food as a society, and food-related get-togethers are common (potlucks, barbecues, picnics, etc.). But it's important to remember that a lot of people may feel excluded when activities revolve around food. We aren't alone. People with diabetes, migraines, bipolar disorder, Crohn's disease, celiac sprue, and other disorders also may feel excluded from food-related activities. Is it their fault? Are they being anti-social?

No. The truth is that there are many activities out there that will involve more of your friends. Ball games, bowling, a movie, miniature golfing, karaoke, amusement parks, board game nights, swimming parties… These are just a few ideas to get you brainstorming. (See chapter seven for many more.)

By taking the focus off food at get-togethers you'll be helping everyone feel more normal without facing the dangers of getting sick. In addition, your eating limitations will not stick out unless you want them to! (If you host the party, try feeding everyone some of your allergen-free food and see what they think!)

I feel that part of getting people to understand is to help them realize that there are things to do other than eating. Food-related parties are great, but when they cause you to leave out some "special" people, they aren't that great after all.

Acquaintances

In a small survey at FAST (with 25 participants), 36% of respondents said that the hardest people to explain their food allergies to were new acquaintances (relatives get the silver medal at 28%). When you're at a party, for example, you may be asked by a fellow guest why you're avoiding the buffet. Do you explain? Or just say you're not hungry?

If people ask me to eat, I almost always have a different response. I don't even consciously think about it, but a few of the excuses I have thrown out are: "I can't," "I have food allergies, and "No thank you." I've never thrown out a white lie, because I know that it could come back to haunt me later.

That might sound like a pretty strange thing to say, but it's a practical approach. Let's say I am at a party and I am offered a cookie. "No thanks," I reply. "I'm on a diet." That's somewhat true; after all, I'm on a medical "diet" of sorts. However, this comment could be taken and turned into a joke at the party. "Look at Melissa! She's skinnier than I am and she's on a diet!" Or, if your excuse is that you're not hungry, you may still be offered food again and again throughout the progression of the evening. After all, you just weren't hungry *at that moment*. You will likely be offered food again.

I find the best route in this type of situation—if there is time—is to offer a quick explanation. In one of my classes the students brought in a donut for my table to split. I said, "Don't leave a piece for me. I have food allergies." They weren't offended, and didn't ask me a single question. Instead, I'm sure they were delighted to get a larger share of the donut than they would have otherwise.

If I am not going to be at the event for a long time, or if food is not the main focus, I typically just say "No thank you," or "I can't." I don't think it's necessary to explain to each individual I meet about my food allergies. As long as eating is not a large part of the get-together, there's really no reason, and it feels great to not have the allergies become the focus of the get-together.

However, there are other instances when I do feel it's important to tell. I had one professor who had put a lot of effort into making a special ethnic dish for our class. She told us all that since she had put forth so much time into it she expected all of us to at least try one bite. Unfortunately, I happened to be at the beginning of the row, and she offered the bowl to me to pass around. "I don't want any," I said brusquely. I even refused to touch the bowl. Immediately, I felt terrible. My teacher had done something nice, had asked us each to take a taste, and I had not wanted to explain to the class about my food allergies. I ended up hurting someone's feelings instead.

After class, I waited to speak to her and apologized for my response. I realized that my response had been because I was trying to protect myself from embarrassment and from having to speak to my class about food allergies.

The next semester, there was a similar situation with students bringing in ethnic foods for the entire class to eat. This time, I explained to the professor early on that I would not be able to sample classmates' foods. Did I feel embarrassed? Yes. But I also wanted to make sure that people knew I was not avoiding their cooking. It's very easy to hurt people's feelings when you refuse something they have taken the time to make. In this type of situation, I believe it is very important to take a few moments to explain, even if you are self-conscious.

Many people are proactive in their approach to explaining their food allergies. They use every opportunity to explain to anyone they meet about their diet limitations. Although I find this commendable, it can also be construed by others as if you are proud of your food allergies or obsessed with talking about them. It is exceedingly difficult to find a "happy medium" between coming across as informative and coming across as obsessed. I think this is a learning experience, and something I am still trying to find a standard for. In some ways, I'm playing by ear from circumstance to circumstance.

One of the best and most noninvasive ways I have found to spread the word about food allergies is to write a report about them for school. I wrote a fiction story for a college class that was about a girl with food allergies. I ended up receiving a lot of questions from classmates who read it. They didn't care for my story, but they had never heard of the condition and were extremely interested.

Anyone who is still in school—grade school through college—has an effective and easy way to spread the word about allergies to acquaintances, *and* reach a large audience!

Friends and Family

Now we've dealt with acquaintances—those that we don't know very well. Yet, it can be just as difficult to explain your food allergies to friends and family. They are people who have known you much (or all) of your life. It may suddenly be difficult for them to grasp the fact that you have an illness. My close friends, for instance, didn't even remember that I had been sick growing up.

My parents *did* remember my various illnesses, because they had had to take me to the doctor and pay for various prescriptions. However, because I was a minor at the time of my diagnosis it was up to my folks to decide what the course of action would be. My mom decided that food allergies were something that could be cured, and took me to get nontraditional treatments. One of the treatments involved ingesting an allergen of mine. For a long time my mom also had me "challenge" my allergens and try new foods, only to see me getting sicker and sicker and missing out on semesters of school. I will admit that some of this was due to my own lack of knowledge about my allergies. For example, I felt cheese was not dairy, and though my allergy to milk was off the chart, I continued to consume it unsuspectingly.

Family members want to think the best. "When will you get over your allergies?" is not an uncommon question. Because of this, family members and friends will suddenly become excited with anything on TV or in other media that is even remotely about your condition. This can be great if they are finding information that is true. But many of the articles, books, and shows that I have been referred to about food allergies are ones I know to be inaccurate. I don't know what to say in reply. After all, whoever told me about it was trying to be helpful. I don't want to hurt a friend by pointing out the mistakes. On the other hand, I don't want my friend to believe what s/he reads or sees when I know it is erroneous! As you can see, dealing with friends and family is a very complicated issue. It is easy to hurt feelings and to have misunderstandings over even small things. Just remember that the intentions of others when trying to research about your condition are good. You may not like the message, but you have to love and appreciate the messenger, because s/he is trying to be helpful.

Another problem with family members and friends can be that they simply don't believe you. Someone might say, "Well, you didn't have the food allergies yesterday. Where did they come from?" I can trace my symptoms back as far as I can remember, but some adults are diagnosed later on in life and don't remember having unusual symptoms growing up. If this is something you experience it can be beneficial to show a doctor's diagnosis and perhaps even tell them the doctor's credentials. It seems silly to have to try and prove something to family and friends, but it can be done in a positive, kind, and educational way. (Don't ever do this in an abrupt manner, which can be seen as confrontational.) What you perceive to be "strange" behavior from friends and family members can sometimes be attributed to the fact that they feel helpless and don't want you to be sick. Sometimes this forces them to deny a condition exists. It's important to realize that you shouldn't get mad with someone who initially has this sort of reaction. Denial can be a pretty common response.

Will you have friends abandon you after you are diagnosed with food allergies? It is likely. When I became extremely ill right before my diagnosis, and had to drop out of school, I wondered suddenly where my friends had gone. No one called to ask where I was (I later found out a couple of them had asked in the office), or sent me a card, or anything. What I tell myself now is that people have lives and are busy with other things. It is difficult to have a friend who has problems, because suddenly my problems also concern my friend. My friend, for example, can't split a pizza with me or ask me to go grab a burger. Being around me is a hassle. It sounds mean, but it's something I have accepted. People who want to be friends with me have to make an extra effort. This sounds negative, doesn't it? But I've got something good to report. The few friends that I *do* have are real, genuine friends. They are people who are caring. They're people who have stuck by through thick and thin. I think food allergies, in a way, are a blessing as far as friend finding is concerned. My food allergies are my "friend filters." I can't maintain friendships with people who only want someone to eat at a pizza joint or donut shop with when they have nothing better to do. I may have fewer friends, but the ones I have are ones worth keeping. The people who don't want to be my friends because of my health problems are not the types of people I would want to hang around with, anyway.

Taunting

Being taunted by people is a whole other ballgame. I don't mind it when someone doesn't want to be buddies with me due to my allergies, but when it progresses into something else, it's not acceptable.

When I was a teenager in school one of my classmates noticed my excessive absences and my generally unhealthy appearance (which has since, for the most part, disappeared). She got up in front of the class and loudly proclaimed, "You have AIDS, don't you?"

Instead of getting angry, I said calmly, "No. I have food allergies."

That same year another girl made fun of me when I had to meet with the school counselor due to my health problems. This student thought the counselor was a teacher who had interrupted our class because she wanted my help, and the student jeered at me for being a "genius." Instead of getting mad I told her the truth—that the woman was a counselor I needed to speak to because of a health problem. This time, the quick comment progressed into my entire class peppering me with questions about food allergies.

As you can see, I try to take something that could be perceived as negative, and turn it into a positive. Some people tease because they simply don't understand. At times snide remarks are how a person asks a question, though they come out incorrectly or tersely. I feel the first girl wondered why I was sick frequently. She didn't know how to express this in a friendly manner, so she instead made fun of me, knowing it would provoke a response. I think the second girl just wanted to know why I had to leave my class. The rest of the classmates, who followed up with additional questions, were interested in finding out more about my health problems. (They were also interested in getting out of listening to the teacher's lecture, of course.)

You will very likely be ribbed at times for your diet. People may accuse you of having an eating disorder or other disease, or of being a picky eater. If you remain levelheaded, what began as trying to pick a fight can become a positive way to inform someone about your condition.

I'm Not the Only One

In dealing with others we must remember that everyone has problems. It would be no fun for your friend to listen to you talk about your health for hours on end. The easiest way to picture this is to recall various movies and television shows you have seen. At least one of them probably had an old lady complaining about all of her ailments ("My bursitis is acting up, and oh my rheumatism! Did I remember to tell you about my liver...?")

We need to remember that other people have problems, too. If we constantly complain and talk about ourselves, we can appear to be self-absorbed or as if we are somehow bragging.

Questions, Questions, Questions...

...and more questions. Chances are, you'll be asked a lot of questions. Maybe by your boss, your friend, your mom, brother, aunt, dog...

Being asked questions about your disorder can become very—OK, I'll admit it—annoying. If your experience is similar to mine, the same people will ask you the same questions more than once.

As with the taunting, you can take this in a negative way, or you can take it in a positive way. I try to similarly see this in an optimistic light. If someone asks you a question, it is hopefully because they genuinely care and want to find out more about what you're going through. What you may find helpful is to set aside a few minutes of "question time." Let someone ask you questions for as long as s/he wants, and then move to other topics. The food allergies should not become the focus of your friendship with anyone, which can just turn people off. I have talked about my allergies in excess before, and I have seen first-hand that it can backfire. After a while people will think you are obsessed with your health condition, don't have anything else going on in your life, and are self-absorbed. So education is good, but it must be education without excess.

Then there are the people who don't really listen. They ask questions just to appear concerned, but don't listen to or remember your replies. The next time you see them they may ask more questions based on their misunderstandings of your last discussion on food allergies. This is what I find the most discouraging. No one likes to talk to a brick wall. But, I also try to be patient and answer the questions I'm asked, no matter how stupid I think they are. There is a saying (made popular by teachers) that "there is no such thing as a stupid question."

As a college student I could probably debate this statement, but I jest. It's never advantageous to lash out at someone or tell them their questions are stupid or that they should have listened to you the first time. Perhaps at some stage this type of friend, acquaintance, or family member will begin remembering what you say through osmosis or subliminal messaging or power of suggestion or…

A Friend You Can Identify With

Because you may find it hard to constantly be explaining your allergies to people, it's important to find at least one friend that can empathize with you. I don't just mean an understanding friend. It's important to find friends who understand because they have health problems as well. But you also need a friend who understands because s/he has experienced the very same thing. As author Jonathan Swift wrote, "We are so fond of one another, because our ailments are the same."

When I was diagnosed with food allergies I really wanted to make contact with others who had them. I wanted to talk to someone I could swap recipes and advice with. Never would I have to explain my allergies, my diagnosis, or anything.

This is actually a lot easier said than done. Food allergies are a rare disease, and if you think back it's possible that you won't remember any friends or family members that have ever said they have food allergies. Perhaps you will remember a few people, but they may only be acquaintances or may not be people you would be willing to develop a one-on-one support friendship with.

One quick way to search for people with food allergies is to check with your local hospital for support group meetings. Many support groups dealing with food allergies are for mothers of children with the disorder. However, it's possible that they would still let you participate. It's worth asking!

Then, there's also the FAST website. I created the website with the intention of making it possible for people with allergies to interact with one another. Though I don't know anyone locally with food allergies, I no longer feel alienated. The Internet has become a resource that has been able to make people who live all over the world feel as though they are next-door neighbors. Of course, the Internet itself has its risks, but we will get to those in chapter nineteen.

In the meantime, try to think of a friend who might understand your situation. It may not necessarily be someone with food allergies. Anyone with a chronic disease has likely faced similar concerns to yours.

It's important to remember that the person you pick to be your buddy is *not* a "garbage dump." In other words, the whole point of a support friendship is to support and be there for one another. If the friendship is always one-sided you will defeat the entire purpose of being a sustainer for your friend. In fact, finding *other* things to do (other than talking about your health problems) is a very healthy aspect that should be present in your friendship. You are also putting yourself into a vulnerable position when you choose one person to be your entire "support group." So be sure that you think through your choices very carefully, and only choose someone you trust completely. For this reason, finding an already established support group to join may be a good choice.

My Problem is Not Everyone's Problem

Now that we've talked a lot about our potential problems with other people, there is another very important side to mention. Could we possibly also be doing things to upset *them*?

Educating others is very important, but there is a way to cross the line into public menace. There are those of us in the food allergy community who expect the world to change to accommodate our needs, and for everyone to care about us.

In some ways, that's fine. There are certain things that need to be changed, such as making labeling easier to read for everyone. But in some instances our requests may actually be unreasonable.

Let me give a real-life example. When my church serves communion, I have become sick more than once (I sometimes react to wheat present in the air). Stop and ask yourself, what would you do? There are probably two possible courses of action. One, you could find out ahead of time and not go to church that day. Two, you could confront the church and ask them to serve something else, and/or not serve communion. Which sounds best?

For me, I have decided not to "rock the boat." I feel that my food allergies are my problem, they aren't other people's problem. Though it is fine for me to ask for certain favors due to my allergies (for example, I might ask a friend not to bake wheat near me), I don't feel that I have the right to ask for all of society to bend to my needs. So I just don't show up when communion is served.

There are some people with food allergies who *do* want society to change, and work to change it. It is hard, as I have said before, to know when one crosses the line and is expecting unrealistic accommodations to be made. When one's health is threatened, especially with possible anaphylactic reactions, at times it becomes necessary to request modifications that others may deem "unrealistic."

Asking yourself a few questions about the situation at hand may help determine whether or not what you want to occur is practical.

- *Am I asking for a reasonable solution?* For example, if you're mad while attending a huge potluck because someone brought along peanut products after you requested they not be present, understand that people do not comprehend labeling as well as you do. Individuals that I have been in contact with think "peanuts" and "peanut butter" are two different things, and for some time after my diagnosis I didn't understand that I couldn't eat cheese because I am allergic to milk. If you go to an event where there will be food, then you are consciously going into a potentially dangerous situation. Being in college, I am around students who bring in wheat products to snack on during class. I have never made a request for them to stop. I know they wouldn't understand the concept of what "wheat" is, and my reactions to inhaled wheat are random (and not life-threatening). However, when a teacher asked my entire class to go meet in a restaurant where there was obviously a much higher chance of my having a reaction, I said "no" and stayed behind. Though asking thousands of students in a college to no longer eat wheat is not rational, it *is* rational to not put myself into extreme danger by meeting with one class in a restaurant.

- *Are there no other alternatives?* Before asking for changes to be made, you should see if there is an alternative. For example, in the aforementioned potluck situation, not going is an "alternative." If you knowingly put yourself into a dangerous situation when there were other choices available, you probably do not have much of an argument. This is never an excuse to become a hermit, of course, but you can pick and choose which get-togethers and other social events you go to. However, there are some situations when you may *need* to ask for special exceptions to be made, such as seeking help at your high school or college in order to graduate. This all boils down to the question of whether a change *needs* to be made, or you just *want* it to be made.

- *Am I acting on emotions or logic?* It is easy to get angry with people when they are putting your health in danger. We have to remember, though, that people in general do not know about food allergies. They are not jeopardizing your health *deliberately*. For this reason it is much more beneficial to deal with facts and figures than to have an emotional outburst. The people you speak to may not care to hear, for example, about all of your symptoms. However, they may listen if you mail them statistics on how many people die per year from reactions to their food allergens. Taking time to do your research is impressive, and it also gives more credence to whatever request you are going to make. Writing a letter is a brilliant way to express your thoughts, because you can keep rewriting and reworking it until it makes perfect sense and sounds more objective. You can also have one or more people proofread your work before sending it, to make sure it doesn't sound reactionary and emotional. (When speaking of letters I should clarify that I *do not* mean e-mails. E-mails often get replied to by a webmaster or a customer service representative. They don't always reach the intended person, even if you ask for them to be forwarded.) Using brevity (coming to the point and not going on for pages) in your letter is best, as well. Never attack the person in the letter; treat him or her with respect. As our moms always used to say: "You catch more flies with honey than you do with vinegar." (Actually, I think you catch more flies with a car windshield than with anything else.) If you never cared for your mom's advice, Abraham Lincoln said: "If you would win a man to your cause, first convince him that you are his sincere friend. Therein is a drop of honey that catches his heart, which…is the great highroad to his reason, and which, when once gained, you will find but little trouble in convincing his judgment of the justice of your cause."

Though asking yourself a series of questions sounds like a lot of work, genuinely thinking through the situation to see if your request is reasonable will offer better results than being reactionary and emotional. Having a "cooling off" period in order to think the situation through will make you come across as an expert on the subject, and you will be more respected for your opinion.

To summarize this point, I feel that there are many times when we are knowingly putting ourselves at risk and don't have a right to ask for accommodations to be made. It is important to think over the entire situation and decide whether or not it is rational to expect people to act in harmony with our requests, and then to act accordingly.

3

Strange Reactions

Though I have many of the traditional symptoms that allergists believe can be caused by food allergies (vomiting, abdominal pain, hives, rashes, diarrhea, respiratory problems, eczema, etc.), I also experience some symptoms that are not as widely accepted.

Fatigue

One of the common questions I'm asked by people with food allergies (and used to ask others) is "Does the fatigue ever go away?"

Fatigue is one of those debated symptoms. You'll find some doctors who say you can be fatigued from your food allergies, and others that pooh-pooh the idea. I find fatigue is one of my most common complaints. Even on a good day I get worn out very easily. When I first went to the allergist and explained my symptoms he temporarily diagnosed me as someone with an illness of unknown origins such as chronic fatigue. This is also something people notice very quickly with me. My fatigue, however, is not the kind where you can go to bed and fall to sleep immediately. When I was younger, the fatigue was accompanied by severe insomnia. I would generally be up until around three in the morning, despite going to bed at a decent time and getting up early for school. After getting off my allergens the insomnia has disappeared, but the other "debatable symptom" of fatigue has never gone away.

For those who are wondering what I mean by fatigue, it would probably be a good idea to explain. I've never been athletic, have been known to drop things, and have always needed more sleep than the average person. But on a more basic level, I rarely have much energy. If I do the exact same activity with someone (even a person twice my age), I am always the one who tires first—whether it be playing badminton, going to school, or climbing stairs. It may sound like I'm just the typical out-of-shape person, except for the fact that I exercise daily, and even the most mundane task is apt to wear me out. My fatigue can get to the degree where I will black out or pass out if I don't stop and take it easy.

Whether or not this is allergy-related could probably be debated. There are other diseases that can cause fatigue such as anemia, certain vitamin deficiencies, and depression, which should be investigated and ruled out. However, I have noticed this trend among adults with food allergies. Is it due to not getting enough vitamins? Or what?

I've had various blood tests to find out what is wrong with me, and they always come back normal (unless they're food allergy tests, that is). So the only thing I have found to attribute my fatigue to as of yet is food allergies.

Unfortunately, despite religiously avoiding my allergens I have found that this is the symptom that persists and refuses to go away. (Eczema is the only other symptom I chronically experience even though I feel I am avoiding my allergens completely, and it is not nearly as severe.)

Saying that I *experience* fatigue is probably of no use to you if it is also something you experience. "How do I deal with it? How do I get rid of it? When will it disappear?"

I haven't found an easy answer to any of the above questions. After being on an allergy-specific diet for nearly ten years, I still experience low energy. Instead of focusing on when I will get over it, though, I try to focus on how to live *with* it.

I've accepted the fact that the things I do must be done a bit slower than other people. It feels very strange to be a "twenty-something" who is still in college, for example, but what matters is that I'm *trying*. It would be so easy to give up, to give in to the fatigue. However, I attempt to do all that I can and to keep "pushing the envelope" to the next level. In college I began by taking a few credits, went down to two, then none, and have finally worked myself back up to eight per semester. I was even able to take a summer class one year. The best that I can do is to keep trying; to keep living to the best of my ability and not let my food allergies get me down. Despite the fatigue I experience, I still feel life is worth living…it is something I would not want to sit and watch pass me by.

Depression

Depression is also another debated symptom. (This may not necessarily be characterized as clinical depression, but rather general feelings of melancholy.) Although at this point this is not considered one of the traditional reactions, I experienced it. My diagnosis came when I was a teenager. I had to watch friends move a year ahead of me in school, miss out on my graduation, etc. Although depression may not be a symptom in and of itself, it is very possible that it is a result of the very different way of life people with a health problem experience. When a person feels set apart or different in any way it is only natural to develop feelings of dejection.

My depression was so bad that I didn't feel like living. Though I was not suicidal, I would sit in the fetal position, crying. The diagnosis and life changes were a shock, and because I have *multiple* food allergies rather than just one or two, my diet was rapidly limited and I felt very different indeed.

It is not a weakness to get counseling. It is actually showing strength. If you feel that you are depressed for more than just a short time, it is a very good idea to seek professional help.

Irritability

Another less-accepted symptom is irritability/grumpiness. Whether or not this is an actual symptom, I won't even offer a guess. However, I believe people can become irritable when experiencing an allergic reaction. When people are sick it's rather unusual for them not to be cranky.

If people don't believe you experience this, ask them how they act when they have a cold or the flu. It's hard to be happy when you're feeling poorly. Then again—if you ask most people how they behave when they're sick, you won't get an honest answer. Maybe you will have to ask their families!

Other Symptoms

There are many other symptoms people claim are caused by their allergies which are not yet well-accepted or documented. Such symptoms that I experienced included daily migraine headaches, general body pain, and insomnia. The good news is that after I got off all of my allergens completely, all of my symptoms vanished except for my fatigue and occasional eczema (a skin condition). Whether or not these symptoms were directly related to my food allergies, I no longer experience them on a regular basis.

4

Making Food Fun Again

The diagnosis of a disease can hit you like a brick (ouch!). Suddenly your entire lifestyle must change. In fact, you may feel like your day-to-day existence completely revolves around your health problems, and that they consume your every thought.

The trick to making food allergies tolerable is to try and create a game out of them. By this I don't mean that suddenly everyone is going to be jealous of you because you have those "fantastically fun food allergies." However, there's a very overused saying that goes something like this: "When life gives you lemons, make lemonade."

What? Did you say you're allergic to lemons? Well then, how about making limeade? Or appleade? Pineappleade? Without further ado (or corny jokes), this brings us to our very first way to try and make your allergies a little more tolerable…

Be a Detective

Is there a pre-made product in the store that you would love to try if not for one or two forbidden ingredients?

Many people do not realize that ingredient listings are non-copyrightable. Although recipes themselves are protected, ingredient listings on prepackaged products are not. This is a blessing to those of us who have food allergies. What this means is that you are free to try and make a recipe by looking at an ingredient label on a product.

One of the things I've found myself doing a lot is what I like to call "detective work." (Just call me "Sherlock: in the Hound of the *Baker-*

villes.") I take a product's ingredient list and attempt to duplicate it into recipe form. People are amazed that I can go on so little information and come up with a recipe that tastes pretty much like the original product. Almost every time, it's "perfect" on my first try. I'm not bragging here (I hope!), because it's actually pretty easy to do. You just have to gather up all of your confidence and plunge right in! I hope my instructions will help you be able to not only make recipes, but to also be able to try *new* things (including those products that contain just one forbidden ingredient—get rid of it by making substitutions in your recipe!)—*and* save money!

Let's begin by showing an example.

Here is a fictional ingredient list, based on the actual ingredient list I used for my salsa recipe:

◆ ◆ ◆

Ingredients: water, tomato paste, green chili peppers, jalapeño peppers, vinegar, sugar, citric acid, spices, natural flavoring, dehydrated garlic, guar gum, salt, onion powder.

◆ ◆ ◆

To begin creating a recipe, I write all of the ingredients on a piece of paper in the order they appear on the label. In ingredient lists whatever is in the product the least is near the end of the list. In other words, the ingredient list is in descending order of what is in the product. This is important to remember when creating a recipe. For example, you would not put in more salt than you would vinegar. Begin by writing down all of the ingredients, and making substitutions where necessary. I give an example according to my allergens below:

- water (No allergy here.)

- tomato paste (I can have this.)

- green chili peppers (I can have these, too.)

- jalapeño peppers (I'm not allergic to them.)

- vinegar (I change this to "apple cider" vinegar.)

- sugar (No problem.)

- lemon juice (When an ingredient list uses citric acid, I've always used lemon juice as a substitute.)

- Notice that "spices" and "natural flavoring" are nonexistent in my recipe. These are ingredients that, by current US law at the time this book was published, can be left off a label. In other words, though these are actual food ingredients, they aren't identified on the label. A company may do this to protect its recipe, or because they simply don't know what ingredients are in the flavoring they used. Either way, it's not enough information to go on, so I'm leaving these mystery ingredients out.

- Garlic has also disappeared from my list of ingredients. I'm allergic to it. Since garlic is so far down on the list of ingredients, I see no need to make a substitution for it; the peppers in the beginning of the recipe will be present in high enough quantities to give the salsa the "oomph" it needs.

- xanthan gum (I react to guar gum, so xanthan gum—which works similarly at a 1:1 ratio—is a good substitute for me.)

- salt (Not allergic to it.)

- onion powder (This is fine, too.)

Now that we've gotten this far, everything looks easy. You're probably thinking, "deceivingly so!" However, it's just about this easy to develop a recipe simply by looking at a pre-made product's ingredient list.

Remember again that everything is in the product in descending quantity. I often like to try starting with around one or two cups of my first ingredient. Then I "instinctively" just jot down smaller and smaller quantities for the other ingredients. I do this all on paper without even lifting a spoon or getting out a bowl!

After thinking it through, I have a finished recipe to try:

◆ ◆ ◆

1 cup water
3/4 cup tomato paste
4.5 oz. can green chili peppers
1/4 cup jalapeño peppers
1 tablespoon vinegar
1 teaspoon sugar
1 teaspoon lemon juice
1 teaspoon xanthan gum
Dash salt
Dash onion powder

◆ ◆ ◆

How do you figure out the cooking instructions for your recipe? This may be the most difficult challenge for you, rather than figuring out quantities! Go by what you think it would be. For example, a recipe such as this one doesn't require baking, and is thus pretty easy. You may also wish to look in a cookbook at similar foods for ideas. With cookies and cakes you can "check along the way" using a toothpick to see if the middle of the product is "done."

Here are the instructions I came up with for the salsa:

♦ ♦ ♦

Combine all ingredients in a food processor. Store in the refrigerator.

♦ ♦ ♦

Note that the ingredients near the bottom (the flavorings—salt and onion powder) are present in similar quantities. Also, the sugar, lemon juice, and xanthan gum all require 1 teaspoon. Don't be afraid to have ingredients that are next to one another in the recipe call for the same or similar amounts, even if they come later on in the ingredient list.

If your first try doesn't work out, don't despair. It can take a while to fine-tune a recipe. If you want to duplicate cookies, for example, check in a cookbook to find cooking times and temperatures, and solids vs. liquids quantities to get a better idea of how to formulate your recipe.

There is a saying that "necessity is the mother of invention." If you need to duplicate an ingredient listing and come up with a product, either due to financial reasons, or the product having a forbidden ingredient in it, I think you'll find this project both challenging (or, hopefully, easy!) and fun. I've come up with bread, cookies, nacho "cheese," ketchup, salsa, salad dressing, and other foods that have almost become a "daily staple" for me, and taste like the "real thing." I wish you similar success!

Let Me Grab my Lunch Bag!

Do you remember how much fun you had as a child every Fall on your search for the perfect lunchbox to take to school? Even if you hated school with a passion, you probably still enjoyed looking for a shiny new metal or plastic lunchbox. Are you ready to get excited again?

Well, I hope you are, because part of gaining back your freedom is being willing to go lunchbox or lunch bag hunting.

It's easy for most people who are out on a trip—even just a day-long trip—to pop by the local hamburger joint, roll down their car window, and ask for a burger and fries. However, for those of us with food allergies fast food can be impractical and downright dangerous. Are you sure you can have that burger? It might have been fried on the same griddle as fish. The fries might have been fried in something you're allergic to; or even contain hidden flavorings to "boost" their taste. Something as simple as a beverage could possibly contain different ingredients than what you would expect, because they are often finished by restaurants from an original syrup form.

That's the *bad* news. The good news is that you don't have to stay inside of your house just because you can no longer get a burger on the go. One way to reclaim your freedom is to purchase an insulated lunch bag. Finding a bag that you enjoy and that will be your new buddy and key to freedom can be a fun adventure.

I found a bag I liked through looking on the Internet. It's shaped like a brown paper lunch bag, but made of insulated material. More recently I purchased a larger bag that I had custom imprinted. Don't despair if you can't find a bag you like. It's possible that a printing company near you (or online) offers lunch bags on which they can put a special photo, or even your own artwork. Imagine having an image of your favorite child, grandchild, puppy, or even your very own painting on a lunch bag. It sounds expensive, but my custom-printed bag cost less than twenty dollars. This is a small investment for how much use you will get out of it.

It may sound silly to call the bag your new "friend." However, this is how many of us with food allergies feel about something that helps make life more normal and gives us more freedom. Now when you go somewhere you can stock your bag with safe snacks, drinks, or even a full meal!

5

Allergists, Doctors, and Medications

Allergists and Doctors

One thing that can be very discouraging for people with chronic, undiagnosed problems is that doctors do not always take the time to find out what is wrong with them. They may tell parents that a baby is just high-strung and crabby. Or tell them that she has the flu when her temperature is actually abnormally low (96.0). Or, they may write a doctor's note for a high school student that says, "she was sick, but she'll be back to school tomorrow," forcing her to attend school even when she feels miserably ill. All of this happened to my family. None of it should have.

Doctors have a lot of stress on them, no doubt. They have to look at many people a day and decide what is ailing them in a very short amount of time. Often they have to base their diagnoses on what their patients say, rather than what the doctors can see (if the problems are not visible).

I believe that ultimately doctors are somewhat responsible for the ill health I experience to this day. Despite regularly going in for checkups, for years no one was able to diagnose me or help me, and my condition worsened with time.

Still, doctors are also responsible for our good health, such as administering vaccines and treatments for cancer and other diseases and disorders. I understand the importance of going to a doctor—the fact is that we just need to shop around until we find one who will listen to our complaints and take them seriously, and take the time to work to find the answer. I will not stop visiting a doctor just because doctors cannot help me "get over" my food allergies. They have helped me with many other illnesses I have had over the years, and continue to do so.

It would be easy for me to mistrust doctors after being misdiagnosed and undiagnosed for sixteen years. However, my health would suffer greatly if I did such a thing. The lack of easy answers—the lack of a quick diagnosis—can be attributed to the fact that I have a rare disease. Rather than blaming people, I must blame the difficult-to-discover condition. In the past doctors have correctly diagnosed me with maladies such as tendonitis, sciatica, a slipped disc, broken ankles, ear infections, and bronchitis, and have helped me with treating these various conditions. Their help has been invaluable to me, and without medical care my quality of life would be lessened substantially.

People who suffer from serious food allergies inarguably need to be under the care of an allergist. Allergists can prescribe medications, epinephrine, and special food formulas. Doctors can also be valuable in dealing with schools. When I was diagnosed with food allergies my allergist wrote my school a note telling them that they should help me with my schooling. Without this note my school would not have believed that I had a legitimate medical illness.

Getting over the Allergies

There are a lot of books and websites out there that say you'll get over your allergies through avoidance, and that they are only temporary. There are still other books that offer a game plan toward recovery, claiming that doing certain rituals or "treatments" will cure you. This type of book sells very well. However, it also leaves people disappointed and disillusioned.

I don't make those claims.

From what I have read on the FAST mailing list children can outgrow many of their allergies, but there are certain foods that one generally does not outgrow an allergy from. Still others say that once allergies are present in adulthood, they are not "outgrown." I won't make claims about it either way, because I simply don't know.

Personally, instead of having fewer and less serious reactions after avoiding my allergens, I have found that my reactions when I have "challenged" my food allergies are much more severe. Sometimes I have ingested a very small amount of an allergen by accident (such as through medications, which will be discussed later on in this chapter), only to find myself having my most severe reaction ever.

I do not plan on being cured of my food allergies. Instead, I concentrate on finding ways to make living with them more tolerable—to accept them and learn to live with them. Having this type of mindset helps me concentrate on today and how to make my life better under the present conditions in which I must live. Because of this, if a cure or treatment is ever found—or if I ever get over my food allergies on my own—I will be pleasantly surprised.

Some people expect the medications they take to help them "get over" their allergies. However, medications themselves (at this printing) cannot cure food allergies, and can even be the *cause* of allergic reactions.

Ingredients of Medications

If you are like many patients, you've gotten complimentary drugs from your doctor before that don't contain ingredient lists. Or, you have purchased medications and vitamins without understanding what certain ingredients are—or haven't even been able to find an ingredient list to begin with.

Well, here's the bad news. Even prescription medications intended to relieve people of their allergic symptoms often contain common allergens! Here are a few of the food products frequently found in allergy medications: citric acid, corn, fruits (various), gelatin, milk, potato, unspecified flavoring, unspecified starch…and that's just the beginning.

Sadly and surprisingly, even your druggist, doctor and allergist may not know that food ingredients are present in medications. For example, when I went to pick up a prescription the woman fulfilling it told me that a generic version of a certain painkiller would only have pain medication in it (of course, it didn't). I knew she was wrong, but she didn't believe me when I tried to explain that medications are not simply and exclusively drugs. When I told another druggist who asked what my allergies were that I had food allergies, he gave me a dirty look and said, "not *that* kind," as if they were totally immaterial.

People with serious food allergies can react to minute amounts of their allergens, and I have personally found that even the small amount present in medications can have an effect. Over the Christmas holiday of 1997 I was prescribed two prescription medications. I had been prescribed them before and had experienced a reaction, but I figured it was only some sort of mild drug side effect and that I would get better over time (though I have never reacted to drugs themselves before). The second time I was on these drugs things went much worse. On Christmas Eve I was seriously stricken with chills, diarrhea, shakes, and vomiting.

I removed myself from the medications (they were trial medications and I was not required to remain on them) and all symptoms subsided. I investigated on the Internet and learned that one of the drugs contained lactose, which is milk-derived, and I am severely allergic to milk. Our family doctor had never mentioned that food products were present in this drug, and since he had given me free samples, no package inserts (or lists of ingredients) were at my disposal. I became so ill as a result of this lack of available information that I missed half a semester of school. That is why I feel it is so important to share this information with others.

There are various ways to learn about the ingredients of your medications if you are unable to find them prominently displayed on your prescription. (Which is most likely bound to be the case!)

I have found that with brand-name prescription drugs, often just typing in the drug name with a .com in the form of "[drug name here].com" in my web browser points me straight to the drug's website on the Internet. I then have to do a lot of browsing within that page for the ingredient listing, sometimes listed under "package insert" or near "chemical make-up."

Package inserts are one of the easiest ways to find ingredients. A lot of people throw away these long lists of side effects and chemical make-ups without realizing the very information they need to know is also hidden within all the technical information. Check this package insert for the term "inactive ingredients." This is generally listed below "active ingredients," which is often by the chemical structure (drawing).

Your physician is another resource. Doctors can pre-check ingredients using a physician's reference (book) or Internet resource. However, there is a huge drawback to asking your doctor to check. I had a doctor do this for me during a visit to the ER for a severe ear infection. She worked very hard to find a suitable antibiotic, but when I went to pick up the prescription the pharmacist switched it on me. Pharmacists often switch prescriptions, giving patients generic versions of the medication, or a similar medication from a different company. The inactive ingredients in generic/similar versions of medications can vary. They may do this as a favor to save you money, because your insurance company requires it, or because they don't carry that specific brand. However, it is not necessarily a favor when you have food allergies.

While reading the list of inactive ingredients you may have noticed some non-recognizable ingredients within that listing. Things such as caramel, flavors and starch may also possibly be your allergens, but they aren't specified clearly enough for the average consumer! If you noticed these or similar terms listed you may wish to contact the company further to find out exactly what they are.

Health food supplements, which many people turn to in an effort to ingest a sufficient amount of vitamins, often contain lists of what they *do not* contain rather than what they *do* contain. There are two problems with buying this sort of supplement.

First of all, these supplements cannot be trusted to be 100% free of what they claim they are, since products may be cross-contaminated, or the labeler may not have known that xanthan gum, for example, can contain corn. As a rule, I never trust labels of this sort.

Secondly, all of your allergens may not be listed. Say a medication claims to be free of your allergens milk and peanuts. That's great, but hey—it might contain your worst allergen (let's say it's wheat). This type of labeling is confusing and not very helpful.

Because of this, and because I have multiple food allergies, I make it a rule to only trust vitamins that contain a complete listing of what *is* in them, not what *isn't*.

Also be aware that health food style supplements are not regulated as drugs, but rather as foods. They may not contain any active ingredients whatsoever. My father, who is a scientist, ran tests on a supplement he wanted to take. He discovered that it didn't contain the active ingredient. This has also been discussed on the national news (ABC news 8/4/99 had a segment in which they covered this topic.)

Unfortunately, we don't all have labs or investigative news reporters around to find out more about the supplements we take. However, you should be aware that the supplements you rely on for vitamins may not contain the vitamins they claim to. It is important to strive for a balanced diet and to get your vitamins straight from the best source—the food you eat. Speak to your allergist or doctor and work with him or her to find out if you need a multivitamin in your diet, and then work together to find one that is safe.

Please remember that nearly every vitamin, pill, and prescription medication will have *inactive* ingredients in it! These inactive ingredients are derived from foods. Inform your doctors about this possibility so that they can help you in your quest to avoid your allergens.

In addition, never remove a prescription medication from your diet without first consulting your physician. The results of stopping a prescription without first inquiring with your doctor can be catastrophic!

6

Eating Out

After reading chapter four (about buying a special lunch bag) you may have started wondering, "Doesn't she *ever* eat out?" The answer to that question is "no." Though this is a completely personal decision, I feel that I am making it based upon research and past experience rather than on emotion.

I have gotten sick too many times after going to a restaurant to make it worth the effort or chance. Despite trying to be careful with ingredients in dishes, I got sick every time I ate out. (Keep in mind that I have multiple food allergies, not simply one or two. My comments in this chapter are of course geared toward those who have multiple and/or severe food allergies. Someone who has one mild food allergy, for example, may not find eating out dangerous or difficult.)

The *Journal of Allergy and Clinical Immunology* (Vol. 107, Number 1) contained a report about over thirty fatalities that took place over a few years, involving people with food allergies (at the time of this printing the report is mentioned on the Food Allergy & Anaphylaxis website, located at **http://www.foodallergy.org**, under the research section). According to this report almost half of the reactions came about as a result of eating restaurant food or food from other "food service" type situations. I personally read in my local paper of a man who died in a nearby town after eating in a restaurant and being assured by them that his food was allergen-free.

I do not say this to scare anyone into not eating out in a restaurant. However, it is very important to realize some things about restaurant dining.

One of the problems with eating out is that restaurant chains can differ from place-to-place. If you find a local restaurant where you feel safe eating, the same chain or franchise a few miles away may have different ingredients in the exact same dish that can make you sick. This happened to me personally. Two chain restaurants in the same city apparently used different chips, and I got sick at one of the restaurants, but not at the other (I knew the illness was from the restaurant food, since I had an immediate reaction). What they did have labeled (such as their special sauces) was extremely vague. This is what finally convinced me to stop eating out. I decided that the convenience of eating out was not worth risking my health. Different products and/or practices in each chain can cause a problem because, after time, you may develop a "comfort-level" with a specific chain. Perhaps no matter where you have gone…no matter what town or state…this chain has used the same ingredients and cooking practices as the others in the chain. However, you only need to have *one* that doesn't handle food preparation *exactly* the same in order to potentially experience a reaction. Never get into an attitude of complacency when eating out. Make sure you check ingredients and possible cross-contamination each and every time.

Another problem with restaurants is their "secrecy." They may have secret recipes, secret sauces, and family recipes that they will refuse to share. Restaurant chains that do offer ingredient lists will generally not tell you of possible cross-contamination, such as what can occur when different foods are cooked on the same grill. This can obviously also differ from location to location. Still, it is rare that a restaurant will let you behind the scenes to give you a one-on-one tour of their facility and divulge all of their ingredients in an effort to quiet your qualms about eating there.

Also consider the fact that when you find a restaurant that totally understands your allergies and does everything exactly within your dietary needs, the next time you go there a new manager, chef or new waiters might have been hired, and the others promoted or gone. If you do eat out, don't ever assume that the friendly and helpful chef who knows you personally is still working there. Find out for sure!

I used to eat out to fit in when I was a teenager, such as going out with a group of friends for lunch after church. I think eating out is especially a problem for teens with food allergies. At that age we try to be like others and not stand out, so we won't always stop and ask about ingredients and incidental additives, etc. In addition, eating out after church was a very normal activity and a special treat for me to enjoy with my family. Due to both of these situations, I ate out many times even after my diagnosis of food allergies.

Convenience food suddenly isn't convenient, though, when you have the allergies to deal with. Making sure something is completely allergen-free is difficult when a restaurant does not understand food allergies. My mom, who is simply lactose intolerant, has asked for dishes to be cheese-free, only to find cheese present in the dish. One time when my dad ate out he was assured that the dish he ordered would not contain any peanuts, but when it arrived it contained visible pieces of them. When we ate out after my diagnosis we spent a lot of time in the restaurant trying to get orders redone, sorted out and "allergen-free." Even with all of these efforts, I still managed to get sick.

I am concerned that some people with food allergies do not take it seriously that many food allergy related deaths can be traced to restaurant dining. We are only doing ourselves a disservice if we decide to ignore that certain foods can cause harm. I realize that many people with food allergies do eat out. I believe it is a personal decision, but that it should not be done without first thinking about the possible consequences, and coming up with a practical game plan before you go.

By mentioning not eating out, I am in no way trying to keep people from doing things outside of the house. I regularly find things outside of the house to do, such as shopping, church, movies, the zoo, museums, miniature golfing, etc. Not eating out is not an excuse to board yourself up in your house and act like a hermit. Instead, it is important to take this as a challenge and to find fun activities that don't involve food. I've found that there are many other things to do with friends and family. I actually enjoy the activities I have discovered a lot more than going to a restaurant. I don't have too many memories of "going out to eat" that have remained special in my lifetime. Well, I do remember the humorous time I was served an extremely well-done hamburger (it was ashes), but other than that, eating out never built memories in my mind. Conversely, I have individual, wonderful memories of other activities that I have done with family and friends, such as my favorite ride at the amusement park or beating my whole family at miniature golf. I think my food allergies have helped me discover that food isn't everything. Good times with friends and family can be found in a restaurant, perhaps, but they can also be found in other activities. Best of all, I don't get sick afterward! (Chapter seven has many ideas for substitute social activities.)

Allergen-Free TV Dinners

Of course, we don't want to eat out just for "social reasons." There's also a practical reason to eat out. Eating out offers quick food with very little effort. If you're a busy mom or dad or have a full-time job, you probably long for a quick and easy meal.

Unfortunately, when multiple food allergies come into the picture sometimes almost every food needs to be made from scratch. However, there are still ways to make "fast food," food allergy style. Crock-pots are one way to make a convenient meal, but one of my favorites is TV dinners. TV dinners? How?

Have you ever wished you could just pop a TV dinner into the microwave and let it heat up, only to take out a delicious meal that took you minutes to make rather than hours? A few years ago I thought about this problem. Having food allergies, we soon learn that our food takes a long time to cook, since it generally must be made from scratch. But, believe it or not, it's possible to make meals fast and easy.

Everyone groans at the thought of leftovers. But TV dinners are more fun, using cute, special plates, and allowing for family members to pick their own favorite food combinations. They give a sense of normalcy to those who cannot eat "normal" foods. For children, a flat toy can even be placed inside the meal (to be removed before heating) for a surprise, just like "real" children's TV dinners bought from the store.

Finding the perfect TV dinner dish can be a bit of a search, however. Check in department stores (such as ones where food storage items are sold). Find a dish that features all of the following:

- Segmented into three (or more) sections. By getting a sectioned dish, you can freeze a few different courses together and keep different foods from "touching" (which kids—and some of us adults, too!—hate).

- Removable lid. Make sure you test this feature at the store. The easier to remove, the happier you'll be with it.

- The dish *must* include a notice that it is microwave-safe.

- If you have a dishwasher, you will really benefit from having a dishwasher-safe product. This extra feature will make having TV dinners even more convenient.

- If you plan on using it for soups, deep dishes are better than shallow ones. (Note: TV dinners containing soups should be thawed out first, because soups take longer to heat up since they turn into ice.)

Now comes the big question: What goes into each segment? The simple answer is precooked foods (yes, now you have a use for leftovers!). Make sure all foods are precooked, except for things such as canned veggies, which will cook in the microwave.

I have found that it works best to have a dessert, vegetable, and main course (one in each segment of the dish).

If you are stuck for ideas, think of things you normally enjoy eating, and when you cook them be sure to make extra. Maybe a vegetable to put in one segment would be peas, beans or corn. The other section might contain a cookie or cake. Your main course choice might be meatballs, refried beans or a slab of meat.

Meals take about four minutes to heat up, depending on what you're reheating. I heat up my TV dinner for about two minutes, turn the dish, and heat it another two, but microwaves vary. Food gets hot quickly in a microwave, so be sure to use oven mitts to remove the food.

Can't I *Please* Eat Out?!

Many people with food allergies *have* found at least one place other than their homes where they feel comfortable eating. It may be possible that you will find the same. However, I have offered this chapter as an honest account of my experience with dining in restaurants. Perhaps you can learn from my mistakes and locate a restaurant to eat in that caters to your diet—or, of course, you can simply take along your special lunch bag when you go out to eat with others. I *don't* want to leave you with a feeling of dejection. Everyone's allergies are very different, and this is exclusively my own experience. Just remember that when you eat out you can never be too cautious concerning your special needs.

7

Finding Something to Do

It's very likely that you're frustrated and feel that you can't do things that "ordinary" people can. Food is an integral part of many outings and get-togethers. In a survey of FAST site visitors in Spring 2000, with 673 respondents, 85.7% expressed that they felt food allergies kept them from doing "normal" activities. How discouraging! But how true. Most people want to meet over coffee, breakfast, lunch, or dinner when they get together with friends. People who have food allergies may feel discomfited when asked out to eat. Suddenly, going out with friends, on a date, or with family seems like something that will never happen again!

In spite of this, it is very important to maintain your friendships and family relationships. If you find that your allergies make this impossible to do over a meal in a restaurant, there are different ways to spend time with others, and we will get to them soon.

However, if you have been invited to a food event here are some options you may not have considered:

- Take "safe" food along in your lunch bag. Since you've read the chapter on lunch bags (unless you are like my mother, who loves to read books backward), hopefully you have taken it to heart and purchased your little "buddy." Now that you have a lunch bag, you should be able to participate in potlucks, cookouts, and family get-togethers in which food is involved. My philosophy is to always take more than I think I need. That way if the outing ends up being longer than I expected, I won't be without extra food.

- Ask when the meal will be through. Some activities, such as church activities, may begin with a meal and progress into something else. For example, when my church had a get-together we found out when the picnic part of the get-together would be through. I went there after people were done eating. I was still able to go on the hayrides and surrey rides, but didn't have to feel left out or awkward.

- Eat ahead of time. Before going to an activity where there will be snacks, it is a good idea to eat ahead of time. You won't be tempted to "cheat." If you are in a very busy atmosphere and new acquaintances ask you why you're not eating, you have a choice. You can take the time to explain your allergies. If you don't feel comfortable talking about them, you can just say, "no thank you. I ate before I came." Although some of us are eager to explain our food allergies to every inquiring mind, at times you may feel more comfortable not having to explain (especially if it's a hectic/crowded place with little opportunity to).

- If your family/friends want to get together to eat, why not volunteer to provide the snacks? You can even host the party, and show them how great the foods you eat can taste.

- Is your group going to a restaurant, and you don't want to eat the restaurant food? Call the restaurant ahead of time to find out if taking your own food in is okay. If not, you can still go and just ask for a glass of water, and join in the conversation.

Of course, eating isn't the only option when getting together with friends and family. There are many other activity options that can be taken into consideration.

Find a Hobby

Admit it. You know a few people to whom you'd like to say: "Get a hobby!" Perhaps they have nothing on their minds except their jobs, relationships, or children. Perhaps this even explains you.

Finding a hobby sounds like a burden, but it can be fun. The good news is that having a hobby or outside interest is a way for you to meet new people, *and* do things with your current friends.

If you're at a loss for where to begin, try asking your friends what their hobbies are. Do you have a friend who likes to hit the golf course? Ask if you can go along next time. A friend who bird-watches? See if she has any extra gear so that you can go on a search together in a local nature center. Do you have a friend who gardens? Maybe he will give you some gardening catalogs or seeds. Chances are that your friends will be more than happy to share their hobbies with you.

Maybe your *friends* also need ideas for activities that don't involve food. If so, here are a few to get you started:

- Go mall walking. This is when people walk around the inside circumference of a mall in order to get exercise. If you're not allergic to dogs and you or your friend have one, try walking the dog outdoors for some quality time together.

- Check around for museums. Interactive museums are best. They're different because, instead of containing "do not touch" signs, they encourage you to interact with the exhibits. You might be able to play with magnets, climb a rock wall, or even put your hand into a "tornado."

- Window-shopping, which is browsing through department and clothing stores without the intention of buying, is a great way to spend time with a friend who has similar taste.

- Check for local sporting events, movies, and plays held in your town.

- Visit a zoo for a day. Don't forget to take along your lunch bag!

- You're never too old to have a sleepover! Have a "theme night" with a friend or two. For example, a movie night, makeover night, game night, role-playing mystery night… If you host it at your house, you can provide the snacks!

- If it's a nice day outside, there are various outdoor games that are fun to play with one or more friends. These include horseshoes, badminton, and croquet. Lawn games can be purchased for a fortune in many stores, but you can also find cheaper plastic versions in dollar stores that serve equally well and don't empty your wallet, or even make them yourself. I have created two games that I will share here. After playing various lawn games you will probably start getting goofy ideas like mine, whether they be variations on old games' rules, or completely new games altogether!

  - Lawn golf. With a tee, golf ball, and club (putter) you and a friend can spend hours in your yard playing "miniature golf." To set up for this type of game, purchase a small piece of straight PVC pipe, dig a hole, and put it in the ground in an area that does not receive heavy foot traffic. Take turns deciding where the tee should be placed. Keep score, and remember that the lowest number wins!

  - Badminton on a stick. This is a version of tetherball, only it involves a badminton birdie! This game was one I invented after realizing I had a problem. First of all, I had a bunch of badminton racquets, but no net. Secondly, when I played with a net available at the local park I found that my friends and I would spend more time running after and picking up non-volleyed serves than we would actually playing the game. To create badminton on a stick, go to a hardware store and find a very narrow piece of PVC pipe and a long, thick stick (used for replacing handles on brooms) that fits inside of it. Bury the pipe in the ground, and stick the broom in it. This creates a removable lawn game. Add a screw to the top of the pole that has a loop on the end. Tie a long piece of twine to the loop, and tie the other end to the birdie. The rules for playing are exactly the same as with normal badminton, but I have found that only underhanded shots work well.

For more activity ideas you can check with your place of worship and find out what activities they offer. Many times the bulletin will list various activities you can get involved with. Even your phone book will have many ideas in it. Start at the letter "A" in the yellow section and page your way through art stores to zoos!

Be Your Own Buddy

I don't mean in any way that people should become recluses because of their food allergies. However, there may be times when you're feeling a bit sick and are stuck in your house. Is this a time to mope and be depressed because you don't feel well enough to be with your buddies? Well, it could be—but being sad is a waste of time!

It's easy to get caught up in always being with friends and to forget how to enjoy being by yourself when you're sick or your friends are busy. Solitary activities help you take advantage of every minute and remember to take time for a very special person in your life. That's you! Need ideas? Well, good! That's what I'm here for!

- Sing karaoke. If you don't have the money to invest in a real player, you can sing along with your favorite album.

- Start a collection. Think of something you really like and maybe already have more than one of. For example, maybe you like keychains, beanie toys, or US state quarters. Put all of those items together in a display case or bookshelf. Next, work on adding more items to your collection. If your friends and family are told you have a collection going, they'll know what to buy you this Christmas other than argyle socks (that is, unless your collection *is* argyle socks…)!

- Learn a new skill. You'll be a hit at parties if you know a skill that is difficult to master. Some ideas include learning Origami (paper folding), coin tricks, how to play the harmonica, card tricks, how to juggle, magic tricks, how to make balloon animals, or yo-yo tricks. You can find books in your local library or bookstore which explain step-by-step how to master new skills.

- Make a collage or scrapbook of special people or events in your life. If you would like to make a scrapbook there may be classes in your town that teach how to do this artistically. Check with your local craft store.

- Visit your local library or video store to find classic movies that have a connection to one another. Pick a genre (Hitchcock, comedy) or actor (Shirley Temple, Jimmy Stewart) and rent all of the movies (maybe one a week) that they have available in that category.

- Think of an old science project that you didn't do well on when you were in school (if you're not still *in* school—in which case stop reading this book and get back to your homework!). For example, that one where you have to build a bridge made of toothpicks that will support the weight of a shoe. Grow mold on a piece of allergen-free bread (yuck!). If you aren't allergic to eggs, you can try the age-old project of trying to make a container for an egg that will keep it from being broken when dropped from a ladder.

- Prepare for and adopt a pet. Make sure you do your research before adopting. This includes checking with your allergist to make sure there is no allergy present. If you have allergies to animals, a goldfish or betta may still be suitable. One betta or goldfish can be housed in a bowl. Studies have shown that pets do wonders for people's health, such as lowering our blood pressure and helping us deal with our emotions.

- Buy and read a children's magazine. Go to a large bookstore or your local library and take a gander at all of the fun magazines you have been missing out on. Maybe there will even be a few children's books that catch your eye.

- Learn how to play solitaire. Peg solitaire and card solitaire are both great ways to waste lots of time, and don't expend much energy (other than mental energy, that is!).

- Make up new lyrics for a song. For this, you have to be in a very giddy, poetic mood. Making a song parody is a little difficult, because you will need to keep the syllables in a line very similar, or the song doesn't keep the same feel. It's a lot harder than it sounds, and a fun challenge.

- Play jacks. Although this game is supposed to be played by two or more people, it can still be played all by your lonesome. After you have honed up on your skills and become a master at the game, challenge someone you know to a duel. The same goes for playing marbles.

- Browse catalogs. Do all the catalogs you get in the mail get thrown in the trash? Try saving them up for a rainy day. I have a place that I reserve for catalogs. I have to sort through it regularly, though, as these things tend to pile up very quickly! I save catalogs for "rainy day" window-shopping.

- Sew. If there is a sewing machine collecting dust in your house, get it out and create something wonderful! You can make hair accessories (if you don't want to have a big project), take up quilting (if you want to be busy forever!)…the sky is the limit! Go to a fabric store and look in their pattern books for other ideas. There may be a volunteer service in your area where you can donate quilts and blankets to a good cause.

- Send a thank you. Is there someone you have neglected to send a thank you note to? Or, is there someone who has made a major difference in your life? Take a few moments to send them a thank you through the mail.

- Invent your own awards for movies. (This can also be done with a few friends.) You could award a movie for having the most obvious mistake, best action scene, etc.

- Learn how to crochet or knit. This is something relaxing that you can do even while watching TV or talking on the phone.

- Invent your own awards for friends, family, and extended relatives. You can print up certificates for people on a computer, or even make them by hand. Ideas include: best shoulder to cry on, biggest heart, and so on.

- Create your own board or card game. You can create a game like solitaire (for one person), or a game that your buddies can also play. Maybe your game will just be a variation on a regular card game, with some new, goofy rules. Make sure you write them all out (so there aren't any arguments), and then test the game with your friends. Be patient, because it may take a while to get all the kinks out!

- Start a journal. Writing down your feelings is a great way to sort them out. There are all sorts of journals people write. A few ideas include a poetry journal, a diary, or a prayer journal. Some people with allergies even have food diaries that they use to keep an eye on what was ingested every day.

- Start a windowsill garden. Find herbs that are safe for your diet, and plant them in a planter. Perhaps you'd rather take up bonsai, the art of miniaturizing trees (which do best outdoors).

- Have a one-person slumber party. Pop some popcorn (or fix a different dessert that fits within your diet), get into your fluffiest, fuzziest slippers and pajamas and sit down to an evening of watching movies or reading your favorite book. Don't tell yourself scary ghost stories—you might not be able to get to sleep! Oh yeah, I forgot. The whole point to a slumber party *is* not sleeping.

- Go to a craft store and walk around, looking at the shelves for craft ideas. They may have kits available for helping people who are new to crafts. Some kits include paint-by-number, jewelry making, model making, and carving.

8

Less Common Allergies

Being allergic to peanuts, milk or shellfish is one thing. Many people have heard of these types of allergies and may even somewhat understand them. Being allergic to something like a fruit or a spice, conversely, is another thing altogether. These allergies are more difficult to explain to friends and relations because few people have ever heard of them. However, it's possible that they aren't as uncommon as we think.

In a survey conducted on the FAST website in 2002 with a little over 900 participants, 75.8% reported that they had what has been termed "uncommon food allergies." That is over 3/4 of the respondents! Obviously, as it was not allergists answering the question and this was not a scientific poll, it is hard to verify the results. However, the outcome of the poll should still be encouraging to those of us with less common allergies. We are not alone. However, since only a small percentage of people have food allergies, it is very likely that you will never meet someone else with your rare allergy "in person." This can make you feel very alienated. Even worse, it can be difficult to explain to others about your less common allergies, because they aren't discussed in the media as much as the more common ones.

Strange Ingredients

One of my less common allergies is an allergy to all gluten. This means that all gluten-containing grains—which are easier to cook with than those that do not contain gluten—are off-limits to me. Although this sounds like an odd allergy, it is one that I have been tested for through a traditional blood test, diagnosed with, and have "challenged" positive on.

I think part of being able to explain your allergies to others is to be able to refer to your "clinical testing." When I tell people I had blood tests performed that diagnosed me with food allergies, they are much more understanding and believing than if I just say that I have them. Most people respond with, "You had a test? What kind? I didn't know there were tests for that sort of thing."

Contact/Inhalant Allergies

Another less common problem is having food allergies that are so severe that mere contact with them, or even just inhaling them, can cause a reaction. These are even more difficult to deal with than having allergies to less common foods. This is because they can make social situations difficult, and can even be something that pushes a person into forced isolation.

Aside from pushing you into feeling alone, this type of allergy can cause others to assume you are a recluse who avoids get-togethers and other people. It can also lead to feelings of having to defend yourself and your unusual health problems.

I personally can react to wheat if it has been freshly baked. Though my milk allergy was completely off the chart when I was checked for food allergies, the wheat allergy was not very far behind, and seems to be about my most severe as far as how easily I can have a reaction. What makes this even more confusing is that whether or not I will experience a reaction to inhaled wheat is unpredictable. Sometimes I do, sometimes I don't. What further complicates matters is that when I have asked people to refrain from offering freshly baked wheat products at get-togethers, they have not understood what that means. What is wheat? What is wheat in? Many people don't know, and thus I have found that it is impractical for me to ask them to not serve wheat products. I can't rely on others, because they don't know how to read labels.

("Flour" is wheat?) It could be easy to get frustrated at people's lack of understanding. However, I remember what it was like before my diagnosis. I was not a label expert. The only time I read food packaging was to play the games on the back of a cereal box. I realize that it is not realistic for me to expect everyone to understand my food allergies or even *want* to understand my food allergies. In a perfect world, yes. In this world, no. Some people will understand and won't offer wheat. However, when I am confronted with freshly-baked wheat, I cannot blame the cook for not knowing what wheat is. I am responsible for the decisions I make and where I decide to go. I must evaluate the risks involved, and then decide whether or not it is worth taking those risks.

With a severe allergy, it is also of course very important to prepare for an emergency, even if you do not feel you are putting yourself at risk. Speak to your doctor about ways to handle your serious or unusual allergies. S/he may find it necessary to prescribe epinephrine. It is a good idea to wear a medical bracelet in case of an emergency, even if you don't feel your allergies are severe enough to warrant doing so.

Multiple Allergies

Yet another difficult type of allergic condition is to have multiple food allergies. I was diagnosed with this condition by an allergist. My test results showed allergies to many of the foods I was tested for. Life is made quite difficult with confusing labels to begin with, but when you have more than one allergy, reading labels becomes an even more challenging predicament. Finding foods to eat can become a tremendous challenge. Because of this, one's diet can become so limited that a vitamin deficiency is not improbable.

It is important when dealing with multiple food allergies that a person is medically diagnosed with this condition (as with any allergic condition). Other health problems can cause a person to react to multiple foods. For example, a person with Crohn's disease or celiac sprue may also experience negative health reactions to various foods. It should be determined that there is no underlying problem that is causing an individual to react to a variety of foods.

9

Shopping

You will find that shopping for foods is now a difficult challenge. A health food store is an amazing place to start looking…but it's also "a-*maze*-ing." You may feel like you're lost in a maze when you visit. These types of stores are wonderful to shop in due to the availability of "unusual" foods, but they can also be dangerous because of all of the unknown terms you will be confronted with while there. Ingredient names at health food stores can be just as confusing as ingredients in conventional grocery stores (for more on that, see the next chapter).

Positives

Products carried in health food stores can be great for people with food allergies. They generally have less ingredients than foods found in a grocery store, for instance. Ingredient reading is much quicker in a health food store than it is in the grocery store, where you will be forced to read labels that can often contain dozens of ingredients. For example, one brand of health food crackers contains all of three ingredients. Compare this to a list of cracker ingredients in the grocery store, and you will be shocked. Shopping time can obviously be cut down. As with grocery store foods, health food store product labels should be read every time you buy. Ingredients can and do change without prior notice.

Companies whose foods are available in health food stores also use nontraditional grains in their products. Rather than using wheat in a baked good, for example, corn, oats or other grains might be used.

These nontraditionally used grains will also probably be available to you for separate purchase. Though traditional grocery stores are sometimes now beginning to stock grains other than wheat flour, health food stores will by and large have more choices available.

Negatives

Health food stores, unfortunately, are not the panacea for people with food allergies. There are a few things to keep in mind when shopping in them.

First of all, prices are higher than what you would expect to pay in another foodstuff store. As with many other people who have food allergies, you may wish to shop in both a health food store and grocery store, and not buy from the health food store exclusively. For instance, you may wish to buy your produce and any other "safe" foods from the grocery store, and your treats from the health food store. Otherwise you may find yourself needing to get a second job just to pay for your meals!

Some health food stores cater more to their "health-conscious" customers rather than to those with food allergies. This is understandable, and one must keep in mind that the original intention of a health food store is not to cater to people with food allergies, but rather to those who are health-conscious. This means that products you need (such as rice flour, for example) may be discontinued if they aren't considered marketable to the other shoppers. The good news is that many health food managers will be happy to order your favorite products in "cases" from their distributors. They may even give you a discount.

One of the biggest concerns I have with health food stores, however, is the fact that the products sold there often contain such confusing ingredient names. For example, "spirulina" and "semolina" sound very similar. Many of us don't know what they are. They both sound safe to someone who has a wheat allergy. In reality, one of them is simply basically another word for wheat. Can you spot the wheat product? We'll get to labeling later…I promise (if you can't wait to find out, check the following chapter). For now, this example will make it obvious why shopping in a health food store can be just as confusing as shopping in a conventional grocery store.

Another downside is that the books, magazines, and pamphlets that are offered in health food stores are frequently inaccurate in regards to their information concerning food allergies. One such pamphlet from a chain disturbed a FAST site visitor so much that she wrote to me asking how we could get it removed. (I had also read the pamphlet and was not surprised by her reaction.) You don't need to buy or read the information available at the store, and until you have a good handle on what is true and what isn't, you might wish to simply avoid these resources.

Even More Shopping Options

Overall, I think you will find that health food stores are a fantastic place to look for new products to try. Some people with food allergies don't live near health food stores, so they make regular treks to the nearest one. It's worth it! My mother takes an annual trip to visit her father on the other side of the continent. Every year she looks in a well-known health food grocery store there for treats she can send home to my dad and me, with our various allergies. It's a treat to expand one's diet, and a health food store is a great place to look.

There are other sources to check out for specialty foods that may not be available in your local grocery. One such source is a food co-op. A food co-op is very fascinating, to say the least. In a health food co-op a group of people in a town agree to buy products from a specific distributor to fulfill a minimum cost requirement. Food is delivered on a regular basis, such as once a month, to a central location. A food co-op is much like a health food store, except for the fact that it mixes a bit of phone or Internet order into the picture. In addition, you are required to buy in cases or other minimum amounts, so you must consider how much of something you will need for a given amount of time, and order accordingly.

Also, if fruits and veggies are in your "OK list," check your town for a "Farmer's Market." This type of shopping experience is generally somewhat like a bazaar where various farmers set up displays and sell their homegrown specialties. If you do any canning for the wintertime this can offer you a less expensive way of purchasing large quantities of fruits and vegetables.

Another source to check for goodies is on the Internet for web stores which cater to people with food allergies and other eating limitations. Ask them to send you a print catalog, or browse their website online. Be aware that this type of shopping is not infallible. More than once when I have ordered from this type of company I have received a product with slightly different ingredients than those listed in the catalog. This was disappointing, but I had family members to pass along the products to. Nevertheless, be sure to read the ingredients thoroughly on each product when the order arrives, before sampling any of them.

Ethnic stores in your neighborhood may be another possible place to check for goodies. An Oriental market, for example, may have many rice-based products that are useable by people with wheat (but not rice) allergies.

Your local grocery store, of course, is still a place to check for your food needs. Many people with food allergies find that their shopping experience there consists of walking around the outside areas of the store (rather than down the aisles) for produce and meat products.

Caveat Emptor: Buyer Beware

Adopt a healthy skepticism when you are shopping for allergen-free foods. Some foods advertise that they are allergen-free, even when they contain common allergens. One such food our family ordered through the mail claimed to be free of all of my allergens. When it arrived I was surprised to see that it contained two ingredients that I am allergic to. The company claimed that the reaction-causing proteins had been stripped from the food. I was not willing to take this chance. Always speak to your allergist before consuming this type of food to find out what s/he advises and whether or not the claim on the product label is feasible.

I also want to throw out the fact that just because something you find in a store is labeled as "vegetarian," it doesn't mean it is egg-free and milk-free (there are different levels of vegetarianism). I often used to eat "vegetarian cheese," not realizing it contained a milk product. Label confusion leads us to the next chapter.

10
Reading and Understanding Labels

Still puzzling over the spirulina/semolina question from the last chapter? Don't worry—I'll give you the answer pretty soon.

I've seen a lot of magazine articles and chapters in books about label reading. However, not one of these articles has ever said the rule of thumb I'm about to give you, which is really all that matters.

If you don't recognize even one ingredient, don't eat the food.

I used to think it would be practical to offer an "ingredient list" on the FAST website. Members and I listed unfamiliar ingredient names, along with a definition of what the ingredient might be derived from.

For example:

acidophilus=dairy
bran=wheat, oats, etc. (grain-derived)
buckwheat=related to rhubarb, not a type of wheat
bulgur=wheat
casein=milk
chickpea flour=garbanzo beans
durum=wheat
guar gum=made from guar plant seeds (legume)
powdered sugar=typically contains a grain starch
semolina=wheat [The answer to the question in chapter nine!]
spelt=wheat (ancient)
spirulina=algae [The answer to the question in chapter nine!]
white flour=wheat

The list went on and on, and it became apparent that it would be impossible not only to keep the list up-to-date, but also to keep it accurate and comprehensive enough to be helpful. I could fill a book with ways to help you read labels, but again I come back to my rule of thumb:

If you don't recognize even one ingredient, don't eat the food.

This doesn't mean that you won't be able to eat the food in the future. I'm saying: "Don't eat the food *yet*." You should ideally research the ingredients further before you ingest the food. It's very easy to give in and say, "Oh, I'll just try it," and later pay the consequences. Instead, it's important to find out what is in the food so that you are not putting yourself at risk for a reaction.

If you have just been diagnosed with food allergies, this rule probably sounds very silly and obvious. However, once you look at a label you will suddenly realize that there are more products than not that contain very confusing ingredients. Once you look at a label you will see that avoiding your allergens is not going to be as simple or straightforward as you once thought.

I wouldn't be surprised if you were thinking, "This is too strange to be true" right about now. My thinking back when I was first diagnosed was that if my allergens were present in a product, they would be listed right in plain view by their plain names. I had never worried about labels before my diagnosis, so it seemed strange to have to start scrutinizing them now. In fact, when someone told me that there was garlic in all the ketchups he knew about, I didn't believe him. After all, it wasn't listed in plain view on any of the ketchups *I* had eaten. However, I started to believe him after I noticed I was getting stomachaches after every meal when I used ketchup. A call to the company confirmed the presence of garlic oil in the product. Yet, it's not on the label to this day.

Hard to believe, but it *is* true. The ingredients in the foods you eat *are not always listed on the label.*

One of the most helpful ways to find out about what unfamiliar ingredient names mean is to purchase a current college-sized dictionary from a well-known publisher (the little pocket-sized "Webster's" paperbacks available for purchase from dollar stores aren't likely to be helpful). If you look in an exhaustive dictionary, for example, you will find that triticale, kamut, semolina and spelt are different types of wheat.

A dictionary is not going to help you in every case. To investigate for hidden allergens a phone call or letter to the company may be beneficial. Unfortunately, the person on the other end of a phone line may be an uninformed customer service representative that doesn't understand labels and doesn't care about giving out accurate information. One time, when I became sick after eating a sorbet, my mom called the company and asked the phone representative if the product might possibly contain any type of milk product. She replied that it most certainly did not. However, the product itself had a kosher symbol that confirmed it contained dairy (we were still learning about how confusing labels could be at that time). When calling a company be aware that you are not always going to be given an accurate answer. Be sure to ask for someone who knows about labeling issues. Quick answers should be more suspicious than when someone says, "I need to check on that. What is your number so that I can call you back after I find out?"

Some people I have heard from through FAST have said that getting the information in writing is a lot more trustworthy than getting it over the phone. In fact, when they have shared the letters that they have gotten in reply, I have seen that the companies appear to be much more careful in their responses. As mentioned in chapter two, "snail mail" (writing through "real" mail), though slower than e-mail, is time and again a more useful way to get in contact with someone who will actually know the answer to your query. E-mails are often replied to by a webmaster or customer service representative without being forwarded to the proper person. However, since e-mail is quick you may nevertheless like to try it (or a phone call) before writing a letter. Just remember that snail mail is often the best way to get in touch with the right person—and receive accurate information—when you have ingredient inquiries.

I trust companies more when they verify something is *in* a product, rather than when they guarantee it's not. Company representatives do not necessarily know, for example, the various words for milk products, whether or not a product was run on the same line as another product, and so on. You can't automatically trust the information they give you.

For the most part, I avoid any foods that do not have plain ingredient lists. This is a tough stance to take, but I have learned through various surprise allergic reactions that I must be very careful with what I eat. I'm happier eating my "safe" foods and not being sick than I would be if I were eating many questionable foods and having numerous reactions.

Even then, this does not guarantee that I will not experience a reaction to a food. Since products are often processed on the same "line" as others, this is another way you may be exposed to your allergens. This type of problem is called "cross-contamination." Even simple ingredients, such as the flours you use, may be cross-contaminated.

As you can see, with food allergies it can often be hard to find "safe" foods to eat. Keep trying, though, and soon you will find many foods that fit in with your diet.

More on "Natural Flavoring" and "Spices"

In 1997 I experienced a serious reaction to an unlabeled ingredient. This caused me to research as much as I could about current labeling regulations (though this applies specifically to the United States, people in other nations may find similar labeling ambiguities in their own countries).

I thought "natural lemon flavoring" on one product I ate, for example, merely meant that it contained squeezed lemons. It turns out that the "natural flavoring" contains one of my allergens (soy). Another food I used to eat proclaimed it had "natural smoke flavoring." I figured this meant that the ham in the soup obtained a smoke flavor when it was cooked.

Not necessarily.

"Natural flavoring," "natural_____flavoring" (fill-in-the-blank), and "spices" can, under current regulations, mean virtually any natural food ingredient which is used to enhance a product's flavor. I have found these terms to indicate the presence of anything from soy to milk to garlic products.

Efforts are underway by various advocacy groups to make labeling somewhat clearer. However, whenever you see one of these terms on a label—especially if you have severe food allergies—you should ideally *avoid* the product until you are able to contact the company and find out what the flavorings are. Be forewarned that in many cases they either will not tell you because they don't know (they may have bought the flavorings from a distributor) or because it is a "secret."

By the way, this is one section of my book that I hope becomes outdated. These two terms caused me numerous allergic reactions before I figured out that they didn't mean what they appeared to. You see, I *thought* I knew what these terms meant…but I really didn't. This brings us back to our rule of thumb: ***If you don't recognize even one ingredient, don't eat the food.*** "Spices" and "natural flavoring" are two ingredients that you *can't* be familiar with just by looking.

Don't guess, because like me you will probably be wrong. The ingredients are often not what you would predict!

Limited Diet

Some people with food allergies find themselves on extremely limited diets. There are a few reasons you may find yourself on a diet more limited than it needs to be. Ask yourself the following questions if you feel your diet is inadequate:

- *Have I trusted other people's information about labels instead of finding out for myself?* For example, if you're on the FAST e-mail list someone might have said a food product contained a certain ingredient. Often, people are correct. Other times people relay information that is out-and-out wrong, a guess they purport as fact, or you may have misunderstood what they were saying. Make sure *you* contact the company to verify any information you hear or read about their products. This is very important, because conversely many people also pronounce confidently that a product is "_____-free" without verifying their information. There is, for example, a margarine that many claim is soy-free, when soy is actually in the product (but is not—at this printing—listed on the label). Never trust what someone tells you about ingredients. Find out for yourself. In some cases it will limit your diet more, but in other cases it will expand your choices! (You might wonder why people pass along inaccurate information. I don't believe this is done on purpose. As the saying goes, "To err is human…" Since ingredient labels can be perplexing it is often hard *not* to make mistakes.)

- *Has one of my allergens recently been added to my favorite product?* If so, you don't necessarily need to cut this food completely out of your diet, because you can make it yourself! See chapter four for information on how to do this.

- *Am I limiting my diet more than I should be?* For instance, I slowly removed all gluten-containing grains from my diet after experiencing various allergic reactions to them. It wasn't until later that I realized I had been severely allergic to them all along, as had been proven on my food allergy blood test. However, some people do remove more and more foods from their diets without being under the care of physicians. Speak to your doctor…s/he may be able to run some follow-up tests to help verify or disprove new allergies.

- *Do I understanding ingredients as well as I think I do?* I may think, for example, that any ingredient that contains the word "calcium" is milk-derived, and avoid it. (Even vitamins added to fortify a food might be derived from common allergens. Vitamin E, for instance, is often derived from a soy source!) However, this is not necessarily true. Again, be sure to check on any unusual ingredients. Just because a product contains unusual ingredient names doesn't mean you won't be able to eat it in the future. It merely means that it may require a letter to the company in order to find out whether or not you can.

- *Would it be a good idea to seek help?* Perhaps you need help from a nutritionist or allergist to expand your food intake. It's never wrong to request assistance, and it may greatly improve your health and/or eating choices.

- *Have I been on a recent product search?* Never give up on looking for new foods to try! New foodstuffs come out *all* the time. Keep checking co-ops, catalogs, health food stores, grocery stores, and the Internet for new foods. Sometimes when I have felt bad about my restricted diet, simply looking in a specialty foods catalog has been enough to lift my spirits as I find new products I can eat.

11

Allergens in Non-Food Items

Just when you realize that foods have ingredient labels (*I didn't know!*), you will also find that products other than foods also have ingredient lists on their packaging. Food-derived ingredients are present everywhere. Sometimes they are labeled. Often they are not.

Labeled

Non-food items that contain ingredient lists include beauty and care supplies such as sunscreen, toothpaste, soap, makeup and shampoo. I have found sunscreen that contains nuts; shampoo with fruit, wheat, milk, soy, and nuts; and lipstick that contains soy and other food ingredients. You'd almost think they were edible, considering how many food products can be found within them.

Unlabeled

There are also various allergens present in products that do *not* contain ingredient lists. Craft items such as children's clays and crayons may contain ingredients like grains and soy. The back of a stamp can be grain-based glue. Plastic and cortisone can be derived from soy. Ink is widely becoming more and more soy-based, as this is considered more environmentally friendly than the former type of ink used.

The Avoidance Question

I feel like a loon when I go into stores and read the ingredients on the back of a shampoo bottle. I do it anyway. Since I have serious food allergies I feel it is important to avoid my allergens as best as humanly possible, even if I am not being exposed through ingestion.

Regrettably, as has been mentioned, there are products that are not labeled. I have yet to find a stamp from the post office that comes with an ingredient label affixed to it explaining to me what the glue is made from.

My personal decision has been to avoid allergens as much as is feasible. If a product has a label on it (such as shampoo or lip-gloss) and I'm allergic to an ingredient, I won't purchase it. I have previously reacted to lip-gloss after licking it from my lips (which is hard not to do when it's flavored chocolate-marshmallow!). If you don't want to risk licking a stamp or an envelope, you might try ones that are self-stick (like stickers). In the United States there are version of these available for both postage stamps and envelopes.

How cautious you will be when dealing with your allergies is ultimately up to you. However, if you have an unexplainable reaction and don't know what the source might be, keep in mind that it is always a good idea to check those labels—even the labels that aren't on food.

12

When Doubt Sets In

At some point, chances are that you are going to ask yourself if the diet you are on is really worth it. You may get frustrated at not fitting in. Perhaps you will begin missing certain foods and will want to taste them again. You may even simply doubt your test results, due to positive thinking or denial.

When some people feel this way, they begin to cheat (or to daydream about it). "Just a little bit won't hurt me."

I have to admit that "doubt" has happened to me more than once, for all of the above reasons. First of all, I would love to be like everyone else. I wish my life's VCR weren't stuck on the "slow-motion" feature. Sometimes it even seems to be stuck on "pause!"

I would love to be able to go out and grab a burger. If I were suddenly without my food allergies today, I think I would actually go out and get a children's meal. And a pizza…and don't forget French fries. I wouldn't stop there, either. I would also remember to grab a bean and cheese burrito, and…

There were also times when I doubted my test results. However, when you have two positive clinical blood tests it's hard to question the allergies. Nevertheless, at some points in my life I have thought, "Maybe I don't have them any longer. Maybe they have disappeared."

I think I first started doubting the diagnosis only a few weeks after I received it! Most people with various maladies have these types of feelings crop up at times. I think it's perfectly normal, and should not be dangerous unless you act upon it (for example, challenging an allergen without first speaking to your doctor, or getting lax on your diet).

There is, of course, a way in which this way of thinking can become dangerous. Some people hold on to a hope for a cure so much that it consumes them. Rather than concentrating on ways to make life more bearable under present conditions, and instead of accepting how their lives will now be, they spend every moment thinking of the one day when they will be restored to perfect health and be "like others."

At first glance it may seem like these people are being "optimistic," which is nothing less than perfectly acceptable and potentially beneficial. Positive thinking is one thing. Basing your entire life around a hope for a cure is another. If all you concentrate on is one day being cured, you will miss out on what life has to offer you *now*. Food allergies do not end your life until there is a cure, when you will suddenly be able to live again. Food allergies are just a bit of a roadblock. Look at them as a challenge; and challenge yourself to find ways to not let them become the focus of your life. Then your differences will not be as noticeable. You will realize that life can be fun and wonderful even when you have a disorder. Though they may make you sick and make day-to-day living a little more complicated, you are still the same "you" that you have always been.

Attitude Adjustment

People with diseases have a choice they have to make. I can be bitter, or I can take something bad and make it better.

My mother has had cancer four times and her husband has a progressive disease. Her philosophy was once, "Why me?" But very soon, she changed that to, "Why *not* me?" If newly diagnosed with food allergies, it's easy to suddenly feel that it's the end of the world and to try to deny that a problem exists. Being without your favorite snacks—ice cream sundaes, submarine sandwiches, pizza—seems like a huge tragedy that you will never be able to get over.

When I was first diagnosed with food allergies I basically lost all of my friends, began to have problems with school, and began having negative thoughts. I can remember watching an old friend graduating and thinking, "She got almost all Ds. Here I am a year behind and not graduating, and I am a *good* student." Instead of being happy for someone's success, I felt dejected because my life had taken an unexpected detour. Instead of being happy that I was finally diagnosed with food allergies, I began thinking of all the doctors who had ignored my pattern of symptoms and started getting mad at them for it. I could have remained angry with my parents for not pushing doctors to find out what was wrong with me. I could have been livid with some teachers who had refused to supply me with sufficient make-up homework because they doubted I was really sick. I could have been mad at my tutor, who rarely showed up to tutor me.

It would have been easy for me to plunge into a deep depression if I had continued with my mindset of comparing myself to others and being mad at the world. At one point, I had to let go of that baggage. I could not spend my life with these feelings. I needed to move on. I had to accept what had happened—or not happened—in the first sixteen years of my life, and let it go. I didn't want to be bitter. I wanted to be better.

I think that having food allergies has helped me grow as a person. Knowing what it feels like to be sick, I have greater concern and compassion for people in need. I'm the type of friend who is told, "I can tell you things I never tell anyone else," and "You're the type of person I can not see for a while, and feel as though no time has passed."

I know I easily could have turned into someone who hated life. I could have felt like the world threw me a curveball. Instead, I feel as though my differences have made a difference in me—a difference for the better.

Can, Not Can't

Part of learning to live with food allergies and adopting a positive attitude is to focus on "can" and not on "can't."

I used to tell people, "I can't have wheat, milk, eggs, peanuts…" I used to think of all the things I was allergic to and could no longer eat, and feel down about it.

Now I try to concentrate on the good. Instead of telling people what I *can't* eat, I tell them what I *can*. "I can have most fruits and vegetables, all meats, non-gluten grains…"

This seems like a trivial thing to mention, but this has helped me remain positive. Instead of looking at foods that I can't eat and feeling bad, I look at all of the things I *can* eat. From those ingredients I've tried to make foods that remind me of those that I can no longer eat.

I'm not implying in any way that I'm a saint. There are still days when I get upset about my diet and wish I could have something that is off-limits. Having been diagnosed a little less than a decade ago, I feel it is especially hard because I can still vaguely remember how much I enjoyed certain foods. There are also days when I wish I could just be a normal "twenty-something" and not have to worry about everything I eat, or stick out when in a group setting. What keeps me sane in these moments is to find a "little thing." Taking pleasure in the "little things" (as we will see in the next chapter) keeps my "why me?" moments and feelings of doubt in check.

13

The Little Things

This summer I stood by the perennial flower garden in our yard. Many of the plants within it are ones that I planted from seed. Looking at them makes me proud, but I'm also in awe that a tiny seed that was sown can turn into a beautiful flowering plant. As I was standing near the garden marveling at the view a hummingbird began feeding off one of the red flowers, only about two or three feet away from where I was. The hummingbird was so small that it almost resembled a dragonfly. Its wings were beating so quickly that they were practically imperceptible. I stood still and watched him as he darted from flower to flower.

This is an example of a "little thing." If I had not been perfectly still and quiet, if I had been busy and had my mind on other things, I may have never seen that hummingbird.

If you think back to your childhood you can probably recall getting excited and amazed by the little things in life. A green archway of trees spread across a street, the shape of a giraffe in the clouds, snowflake crystals on your coat, and a rabbit nibbling grass in your backyard are all examples of "little things" that probably brought feelings of joy into your life. We all have wonderful memories of our childhoods. Whether it's blowing bubbles, climbing a tree, or planting a flower garden, these are still activities you can enjoy now that you are older. Investing in a children's science, craft, or outdoor games book may be just what you need to jumpstart your efforts.

As adults we seem to rush from one thing to another. We don't take time to marvel at the world around us. By not taking time to slow down, we are stressing ourselves out. We are also missing out on some of the most wonderful things in life.

There are many little things that, if we only took the time for them, would help us keep a positive attitude. What about a hug from a child, a baby's laugh, a prism hung in a window that creates miniature rainbows, a slobbery kiss from a cat or dog, a card or call from a friend, or walking through a sprinkler when someone is accidentally watering the sidewalk?

Basically, this all boils down to learning to take life less seriously and learning to enjoy the little things we encounter on a day-to-day basis. As you do this, you will find yourself becoming more and more optimistic in your life outlook, and won't take things quite as seriously. Perhaps you will even make a list of "good things about having food allergies." The FAST mailing list has thought of dozens!

14

Where Are the Recipes?

Hopefully you didn't buy this book looking for recipes, because there aren't any. (Well, okay, I admit there *is* a recipe for salsa in chapter four, but it was used as an example of how to utilize ingredient labels to create recipes.)

The reason there aren't any recipes in the book is very simple. It is because every time I have seen a food allergy cookbook there is as little as *no* recipes that are of any use to me with my specific allergies. This is incredibly discouraging, and is even more so to someone recently diagnosed. If you have looked through cookbooks catering to people with food allergies you have no doubt seen this as well. My theory is that a food allergy cookbook is a cookbook that mostly is of assistance to its author. (Though if you have only one or two "common" allergies, it could be that one of these books will meet your needs as well.)

In addition to these cookbooks still possibly containing your allergens, many FAST members are of one accord in the belief that the recipe results are sometimes not that palatable. After our family has bought and borrowed over a dozen special needs cookbooks, I can honestly say that there is not a *single recipe* from any of them that is used in our house.

I'd better get to the good news.

My suggestion is to create *your* own food allergy recipe file or cookbook, and I'm going to offer you a step-by-step way of doing just that. Though this project will take a long time to complete and will never be a finished task, it can be looked upon as an enjoyable challenge.

Internet Search

If you have access to the Internet, you have a treasure trove of recipes available to you. Search on food allergy websites for recipes. People with milk and egg allergies also may benefit from searching on vegan websites (vegans are vegetarians who refrain from eating any animal products). Some people with food allergies enjoy trying new recipes from other countries and cultures. You can always add other "safe" ingredients to recipes if you'd like to include more food groups. For example, you can take a previously vegan recipe and add chicken to it.

Remember to document on each recipe where you got it. Websites will typically allow you to save recipes for personal use, in their entirety, and with credit to the author and website. However, they may not want you to reprint the recipe or pass it along to a friend without permission.

I find that the recipes available on websites (and through e-mail, such as those swapped on the FAST mailing list) are more palatable than those I find in allergy cookbooks. Best of all, they're free. If I don't like them, it's no big loss.

If you *do not* have home access to the Internet, don't despair. A local college, university, or library may allow the public to use their Internet connections.

Old Cookbooks

Cookbooks from the 1800s and early 1900s may be of benefit because they generally use more "whole" ingredients rather than prepackaged ingredients. For example, a recipe from this type of cookbook might not call for ketchup, mayonnaise or salsa to be added to a recipe. They use single, specific ingredients more than recipes in today's cookbooks tend to.

This type of cookbook can also be beneficial if you will be canning your foods for later use. There are few pickles and *no* ketchups I can have due to my garlic allergy. Canning is a necessity for making certain foods available during the winter months.

What I Can Still Have

Take inventory of your current collection of recipes. Find recipes for foods that you can still eat without adjusting any ingredients. Put them in a recipe book or file. You may be surprised at how many foods you can still eat despite your allergies.

What I Miss Most…

Next, write down a list of the dishes you will miss the most that contain your allergens. This sounds like torture, doesn't it? Thinking about all of the foods you will miss doesn't sound like an incredibly fun activity. I promise that there's a method to the madness!

The fact is that you can make adjustments to recipes in order to make them "safe."

Here are some of the foods I missed most when I made my own food allergy cookbook, along with how I adjusted each recipe to fit my needs:

- Refried bean and cheese burritos in a wheat tortilla became refried bean and salsa burritos in a corn tortilla.

- Chocolate ice cream was made using rice water, cocoa powder, and a few other ingredients. With added rice water in the blender, this also worked for chocolate milkshakes.

- Hot chocolate was adapted to use rice water, water, and cocoa powder.

- Chicken soup could be made with chicken broth, rice noodles (or plain rice), chicken, and "safe" vegetables.

This is just the tip of the iceberg. Coming up with recipes was a tremendous undertaking, but I only had one major flop, and had never seriously cooked or invented recipes before. I know you can do it!

As previously mentioned in this chapter, some people with food allergies decide to forget their old regular foods and instead rely on a new culture's or country's foods. I could never get used to the idea, because I am a picky eater and had lived for sixteen years ingesting foods considered "normal" to the American diet. For me, keeping my diet as close as possible to what it used to be has helped me to be satisfied with it. Having an allergen-free alternative to many different foods has given me the opportunity to feel more "normal." When I hear people talk about burgers, freshly baked bread, and brownies I don't feel quite as bad as I could, because *I can have them, too!*

Check out chapter four for more ways to expand your current food choices.

15

Your Experience Can Change Lives

You have hopefully now learned how to deal with others, make eating fun, create a special recipe file, shop and read labels, and basically accept your diagnosis and learn to enjoy life again.

It is probably at about this time that you will begin wondering how you can give back to others who have food allergies. Or, perhaps you would simply like to lend a hand to people in general. Either way, giving back to people is another way to help increase your self-esteem and enjoyment of life. Helping others can give you a feeling of fulfillment and help you realize your life is for a greater good. Instead of focusing on yourself and your own problems, reaching out to others can give your life a purpose you never thought possible.

The problem is that when most people think of general volunteer work, soup kitchens and food drives come to mind. You may be uncomfortable being around food, especially if it is out of its packaging. Other volunteer work, such as helping to build a house, can require intense physical labor, for which you may lack the stamina. It can be discouraging to want to help out, yet not be able to find an outlet for your aspirations.

Part of finding out the type of volunteer work suitable for you is to ask yourself some questions and see what you're best at. Here are a few questions, along with ideas for volunteer opportunities that should characteristically not involve food.

- *Do I excel at playing a musical instrument?* Check with your local hospital's volunteer center. You may be able to play music for patients and visitors.

- *Do I have a docile pet who likes strangers?* Your hospital or a local retirement center may welcome animal visitors for the patients/residents.

- *Do I enjoy playing with children?* Mentor a child. This one-on-one volunteer job is like having a little brother or sister. Best of all, *you* are typically in charge of the activities and outings, which do not need to revolve around food.

- *Am I patient when someone has a hard time understanding a concept?* Check for child tutoring programs. Similar to a mentoring program, these may be held in schools during school-hours and may not require outside meetings (playtime) with the children.

- *Am I hospitable, well-organized and a natural-born leader?* Consider setting up a support group for people with chronic health problems (or, specifically, food allergies).

Finding your niche as a volunteer is a long process. Simply finding a program you desire to be involved with in your area may take weeks or months (it took me an entire year). Once you discover a program that fits your talents and expectations you will likely have to go through multiple interviews, a criminal background check, and potentially even some sort of medical exam. The time that it takes in order to find a volunteer job and be accepted may be very disappointing and dispiriting. I remember crying out of frustration when I found that I could not do a specific volunteer job that I wished to be involved in. However, I kept on looking and it paid off. In the end, I found a volunteer job that was even more like what I had originally wanted to be involved with.

Don't get disheartened. It may take a while, but the end result—making a difference in others' lives—is worth every effort to get there.

16

Christmas and Other Holidays

Around the holidays is especially when your food allergies may make you feel like you don't fit in. Special holiday treats are just as much a part of the festivities as Christmas trees, stockings, and ornaments. Though almost all holidays seem to have some sort of tie-in with food (Halloween has candy, Easter has eggs), Christmas is the holiday in which many of us probably feel the most left out and tempted to "cheat" by eating the foods made available at the festivities we attend. Which, of course, is not a good or safe option! But the temptation is nevertheless still there.

When Holiday Gifts Are Food

I was in a "Secret Santa" exchange where I specifically wrote that I could have absolutely no food gifts because I have severe food allergies. Nevertheless, I still ended up getting a box of chocolates. Invariably, every year our family ends up getting food as a Christmas present.

When you receive food as a present, your first response may be to feel hurt or mad that your friend didn't remember your food allergies. But before you feel bad, you should ask yourself the following questions:

- *Did I give this person a food item?* Lots of times you will give and get the same sort of gift. People who send a friend a fruit basket, for example, might get a fruitcake in return. People who send relatives money may get money in return. One of my friends and I always gave craft-type/homemade gifts to each other. If you are more creative with the presents you give others, and do not give them food gifts, you will not be sending out mixed signals.

- *Have I ever cheated in front of him or her?* Again, this would send your friend mixed signals. Eating allergen-free versions of things such as cookies in front of your friend may also make him/her think that a gift of regular cookies is also suitable. This doesn't mean you can't eat in front of your friend—just be very clear that what you're eating is different. Even though they look the same they don't taste the same. Let your friend sample your food. That often leaves a lasting impression!

- *Have I been clear enough about the allergies?* If this is just an acquaintance or someone who doesn't know you very well, you can't really expect the person to know what you can and cannot eat. Remember how long it took you after your diagnosis to learn about all of the products that would contain milk or wheat, for example. Some people try really hard to get you something without your allergens, but they just don't know enough about ingredient labeling.

- *Do the holidays make people busy and make people forget things?* The answer to this question is, "of course!" Even your close friends and relatives may completely—and innocently—forget about your allergies in the hustle and bustle of the holiday.

- *Was this food given to me to mock my allergies, or because this person really cares about me?* Remember that presents aren't usually given to be mean (unless you are celebrating your 50th birthday). Although it seems like a mockery to get a fruitcake that contains five of your allergens, the person who gave it to you is really just saying s/he cares about you and your family and wants you to have a merry Christmas.

Now we come to the real question on the minds of people who receive presents they can't use: How do I politely respond when I get a food item for Christmas?

It's easy just to write a normal thank-you, tell a white lie, and say you enjoyed the present. However, this isn't a good idea unless you want to adopt a family tradition of writing white lies! Often people who send food gifts will send them year after year. If you want this type of gift-giving to change, there must be a better solution.

What you might like to do to begin with is to "share the wealth." When your holiday company comes to visit, feed them the product. Here's the key: say, "I got this from a friend for Christmas, but since I have food allergies I am not able to enjoy it. Please help yourself." This does two things. First, it reiterates the allergies. Second, it puts the once useless present to good use and the gift does not go wasted.

When you write your "thank you," let the person who gave it to you know that your guests enjoyed it very much and that it helped alleviate some of your holiday cooking. As an afterthought, you can add that it was so tempting you almost wanted to sample it yourself, but couldn't because of your allergies. This might help in the future to keep this type of gift from coming again. If not, you can always use it on the company. And, hey, that's not a bad idea after all if it's a fruitcake!

Focusing on Food

Some people with food allergies "cheat" on their diets. Most won't admit it, or will guiltily say that they do if questioned about it. And the holidays, of course, are the time when it is most tempting.

I *do not* cheat on my diet. After living for sixteen years where Christmas Eve was unfortunately almost as much a celebration of wonderful snacks as it was about anything else, though, this temptation became especially difficult around the holidays. Seeing my brother eat costly cheese on crackers—his annual Christmas treat—brought me anguish. My stocking on Christmas day—once full of delicious assorted chocolates and various fruit-flavored candies—was suddenly full of *bubble-*

gum. Glancing beyond the lighted tree and across the living room, I could see my brother's piles of chocolates and fruit-flavored candies, and basketball cards! (OK, I'll admit it, I *wasn't* jealous of the basketball cards.)

I wrote to the FAST group and asked, "What do I do?" Almost everyone replied of one accord: "Take the focus off food!"

Since then, Christmas has become more than just a holiday for eating. Although my mom and I have come up with allergen-free versions of various snacks for the three family members on "special" diets, food is no longer the focal point of the holiday. I have found that decorating the house has become my substitute. Following are two fun projects for decorating.

Miniature Christmas Scene Display

Decorate a tree with miniature decorations, including "candy-canes!" Visit a craft store to purchase red and white pipe-cleaners (those fuzzy chenille bendy things that look somewhat like straws, but are not hollow in the middle), and cut them into pieces, about three to four inches in length. Twist the two colors together to make doll-sized candy-canes. If you go to the craft store close enough to Christmastime, you can occasionally find pipe-cleaners that are red and white twists already.

Large transparent beads and safe, small wire meant for putting together flower arrangements make delightfully charming miniature ornaments.

Cover the tree with lights and garlands, and then decorate it with the miniature candy-canes and bead ornaments that you made. Any other miniature ornaments you find in the store can be used, also. For example, our tree always has miniature "gingerbread cookies" on it. Put a doll by the miniature tree, holding an ornament with her arm up, as if she is placing it on the tree.

You can decorate beneath the tree with miniature presents (Styrofoam blocks wrapped up, decorated with ribbons and miniature bows, and glued into piles) and miniature toys. The tree is artificial, the presents are artificial, the candy is artificial—in other words, everything is food free—and it is darling when finished.

For an added treat, wrap 24 real miniature toys and put them under the tree. A child can open one present per day until Christmas.

Children can also help with creating this fun display.

A Village in Your Home

Every year my mother and I go out and purchase a lighted Christmas village building. There are so many buildings available that you may be able to find ones that are applicable to each family member. Adding on to the village every year is enjoyable, and makes for an excellent tradition. If you want to remember in which year each building was purchased you can write it on the base.

To create a display, we use white flannel and cotton for snow on a harvest table. With added decorations and miniature "people," and all of the house windows lit up and glowing—the harvest table seems to come to life!

An added bit of fun is to take one (or more) of the village decorations and conceal it in various places for others to seek out. We hide a Santa and hen in various hiding spots in the village. Children especially love to participate in this game.

Other Holidays

FAST mailing list and bulletin board members have come up with all sorts of wonderful ideas for celebrating holidays without making food the focus. In time, decorating, doing crafts and spending quality time with family may take over as your favorite holiday celebrations. Taking the focus off food can actually be enjoyable!

17

Traveling

If you have figured out how to eat out without experiencing an allergic reaction, traveling is only one step up and may not be much of a concern. However, if you have not found it possible to dine in restaurants, then travel may seem like something impossible. It doesn't have to be.

One-Day Vacation

I do not go on long vacations. When I was younger my parents regularly took my brother and me on trips. I often found myself longing for home. I wasn't doing things I'd *like* to do during summer vacation, like spending time with friends, my pets, and reading. I became even more homesick after noticing a trend when I was on vacations. I almost always got dreadfully sick. I spent our vacation in Washington D.C. relatively exclusively in the hotel room. On a trip to visit some relatives I collapsed into a chair. One time while at a friend's home, I spent much of the evening crying because of a severe stomachache. Another time, at a different friend's home for a week, I spent nearly the entire time in bed. Though all of these examples took place before I was diagnosed, likely they were the result of allergic reactions. I don't know about most people, but when I am sick I want to be *home*.

I still want to get out of the house…no doubt about it. It's fun to get away from the "normal grind" and go on an adventure somewhere else. I pack my lunch bag with safe foods and head on out. Whether it's a wedding two states away or a zoo in a nearby city, I have found that a one-day trip gives me a sense of freedom. I also feel safer in that I have complete control over my food and am only a few hours away from home. I have even been known to take along a bowl just in case I experience a reaction, and always wear my medical tag. People who have anaphylaxis should also be sure to take their epinephrine along, even if only going on one-day vacations. It is always better to plan for the worst-case scenario than to be unpleasantly surprised with an emergency you are not prepared for.

Once you get comfortable with one-day vacations, you may gain enough confidence to go on a longer trip. If so, there are several options you may find physically possible.

Camping

Camping can be a practical way to travel. My parents traveled Alaska in a rented RV. Both have eating restrictions (my mother is lactose intolerant and my father has a few food allergies). With a camper you will have access to a refrigerator and "kitchen on wheels" which you can stock with safe foods. If going far away from home you also may wish to check before you go in order to find nearby health food stores. Your local library may have phone books available for towns in your state. If so, you can call ahead and see if health food stores near or at your destination stock your specialty foods. Also, remember that the camper you rent/borrow has been used by others before you. If you have contact allergies this may not be a viable option of travel. Of course, if you own the camper (and it's new) this is probably not an issue.

Camping in a tent is an alternative, if you take along lots of "safe" food in a cooler, or have food that doesn't easily spoil.

Guesthouse, Vacation Home, or Cabin

If you stay in a guesthouse, rented vacation home, or cabin you will have the freedom and convenience of your own kitchen. As with a rented camper, keep in mind that the kitchens are previously used and, if you have contact allergies, may potentially be harmful.

Cabins *might not* have kitchens. Call ahead and make sure you reserve one that *does* have a kitchen. (Sometimes there is a central lodge where people are required to eat.)

Staying with Friends/Family

Friends and family usually want to help people who have food allergies. They do not want you to have to cook yourself a separate meal, for example, and may want to cook all of your meals.

Speak ahead of time with the person or people who will be making the meals. Ask them to have room available in their refrigerator and freezer for the foods you will be bringing along. Make sure you let them know that you do not want to be a nuisance and don't mind cooking your own food.

There may be a family member (or friend) who understands your food allergies (for example, if you lived with your parents after your diagnosis and they cooked for you during that time). In this type of situation you may feel comfortable trusting someone else with your meals for a change.

Bed-and-Breakfast

Some people assume that a bed-and-breakfast is an excellent place to stay for people with food allergies. (A bed-and-breakfast is typically a home owned by a family where people can reside while on vacation.)

The problem with a bed-and-breakfast is that the person who does the cooking likely doesn't understand food allergies. If considering a bed-and-breakfast, call ahead and find out examples of what types of foods they serve. Some bed-and-breakfasts advertise that they understand how to cater to special diets. Remember that ultimately you are responsible for your own well-being. A claim that the food is allergen-free may not be 100% accurate since most people do not understand food allergies and ingredient labels. In most cases, though this *sounds* like a good option at first glance, it probably would not be.

Motel Room with a Kitchenette

Though more costly than a normal room, a motel room with a kitchenette offers you a place to fix your own meals. This type of room should be reserved ahead of time, as there is no assurance that one will be available when you arrive. You may also wish to check over the phone to find out what is in the kitchenette. It's possible it will only have a refrigerator and microwave.

Remember that the motel room was previously occupied by someone else, and residue from your allergens may exist in the kitchenette and elsewhere.

Pack Your Suitcase or Lunch Bag

No matter where you are headed, be over-prepared. Take along your special "safe" foods in a suitcase (if going on a long vacation) or your lunch bag (if heading out on a one-day trip). Call ahead to find out if stores at your destination stock your "staple" foods. Make sure friends and relatives will have extra room in their kitchens for your meals.

Being prepared—even if you feel it's overly prepared—is always helpful and will ensure a safe, allergen-free experience. Have fun!

18

I'm All Alone

Despite learning how to cook palatable foods, shop, and deal with others, there are probably still going to be times when you feel disheartened because of your food allergies.

While reading this book you may have thought, "wow, this person is a little too cheery for me"—perhaps artificially so. I recently had a friend ask me, "You're happy all of the time, aren't you?"

I'll be the first to admit that I'm not always happy. Those who have something that sets them apart from others or something that makes them different will undoubtedly have moments or days of feeling sorry for themselves. Of course, if any of these feelings persist, professional help should be sought. However, it is also possible to experience momentary feelings of despair due to various aspects of your new "life." Following are a few of the "personal pity-parties" I have been known to experience.

"I'm Not Like Others"

I'm at that age where people are still trying to fit in. Actually, to be completely truthful, I think everyone is still at that age! Knowing my life is not like other people's has been especially difficult for me at times.

When I have complained about this to people, they have basically said to me, "So what? You're different and you're special because of it." My food allergies have kept me from being like everyone else, but they have also given me a life outlook that I would likely not otherwise have. Instead of being self-interested like some people in my age group, I look for ways to reach out to others. Not being like other people can actually be a *good* thing. My life experience has helped shape who I am.

"No One Cares"

When I was first diagnosed with my allergies this was one of the most hurtful experiences I had. I felt like all of my friends and acquaintances at school had suddenly abandoned me. I thought they didn't care. I have found that very few people genuinely think about my health, and it has been discouraging time and again.

What I have to remember is that many people don't understand that food allergies can be a serious health problem that greatly disrupts a person's life. And it may just be my perception that people don't care. In the school example I gave, it turns out two of my buddies had asked in the office to find out where I was.

"No One Understands"

Until you walk a mile in someone else's shoes, you cannot possibly understand what his or her life is like. I don't understand a friend's life the same as she doesn't understand mine.

Food allergies can be an especially difficult situation to explain to people, though, because of how different they are from person to person. I can't expect people to remember all of my allergens, what I can and cannot eat, or what my reactions are. In short, I can't realistically expect anyone to fully understand.

"People Think I'm Strange"

I *know* that some people think I'm making my allergies up. I'm not paranoid—it's pretty obvious. I have what is called a "hidden disability." Just looking at me, most people would never guess that I have a health problem of any sort.

I have a friend who is frequently worried that she or other people will be perceived as "weird." My explanation to her is that everyone is "weird." We all have our own individual idiosyncrasies and quirks that set us apart. Some of us are just more open with ours. Many people spend their lives trying to "fit in" and not be perceived as different. But being different is not necessarily a *bad* thing.

"My Life is in Slow-Motion"

One of the hardest things for me to deal with is my life's VCR. For some reason, it keeps breaking down and getting stuck on the "slow motion," and sometimes even the "pause," features. What other people could get done quickly takes much longer for me, such as getting through high school or college or finding a career.

When this feeling comes into play I must remind myself that I am *trying*. Despite the time that it may take to complete a task, what matters most is to give it my best shot and to not give up until I reach the prize.

Take pleasure in your accomplishments—regardless of how long it takes you to achieve them. Think of how far you have come and how far you can go when you set your heart on something.

"I Wish I Didn't Have to Watch Them Eat Such-and-Such"

There have been many times when I have been in situations where I've had to watch people eat ice cream, hamburgers, pizza, cookies, cheese, burritos…basically, all of my former favorite foods. Although I have allergen-free versions of all of the above, well, you know. They aren't *exactly* the same. Because I wasn't diagnosed until I was a teenager, I still think I have a pretty good idea of what those foods taste like (though I'll never know for sure, and I'm probably wrong since I'm so used to eating my "safe" foods now).

At times I feel like telling people, "don't eat food in front of me unless it's something I can have!" I'm tempted. I don't really say it, though. Maybe I should start an international campaign to outlaw all wheat, eggs, milk, nuts…

I'm just joking here. I have to remember people have a right to eat what they want. Though I will still recall the foods I used to eat with fond remembrance, they are a part of my past and there they must remain. In the meantime, I can watch other people eat them. Watching people eat can be a pretty funny thing, too.

"There Are No 'Real' People"

We are living in a world full of robots and aliens! There are no real people left!

Actually, that's not *quite* what I meant. I'd better quickly explain before you really *do* think I'm strange.

"Real" people are sincere, genuine, honest people. When they say they care about you or ask you a question about your health, you can tell that they care and really want to know. Perhaps you have run into many "real" people. If so, you are very fortunate, and I'm sure you treasure their friendships with you very dearly.

I'm personally the type of person who prefers to have a few close friendships than a bunch of connections to people that I don't really know. Food allergies make this seem more like a necessity than an option, because when I get to know someone enough to be around them to eat, my food allergies can obviously become an issue.

Unfortunately, I do find it very hard to meet people who genuinely want to be my friend once they find out that I'm a person with "baggage." I don't see my health problem as "baggage," but some people do, because it greatly limits what I can do for activities and get-togethers.

Having few friends, though, helps me to see the significance of each friendship I *do* have. In a way, it's simply another blessing. I have more time to devote to the few friends that I have. I have less birthdays to remember, too!

19

Further Resources

It might be surprising to find that the founder of a food allergy site feels that many food allergy resources are not reliable. However, I will say that right now, because they aren't. Anyone can put up a website, and anyone can write a book. Basically, I would guess that most books *and* websites about food allergies are at least partially inaccurate. Even food allergy cookbooks often contain comments and advice that may not be completely correct. I would also be quick to say that, though I have only tried to deal with the lifestyle (and not the medical aspects) of living with food allergies, some may find things in *this* book debatable.

The reason is because food allergies are not fully understood as of yet...not even by scientists and doctors. When you went to your doctor and were diagnosed with food allergies, you might have heard something to the effect of, "I can't do anything for you. Just get off these foods, and you'll feel better." That's what I heard from my allergist.

How frustrating! First of all, I experienced a bit of relief. My disease was discovered, I had something real, it wasn't in my head, I wasn't making it up, and I was going to feel better, and...excuse me? Did you say there's *nothing* you can do for me? But...aren't you a doctor?

Many people are shocked to find out that a diagnosis doesn't exactly mean a cure, or even a treatment, is available. Now that we know what's wrong, we long for quick answers. However, food allergies don't have a "quick answer." Really, your doctor is right when s/he says, "I can't do anything for you. Just get off these foods, and you'll feel better." (I'm hoping that someday soon this statement will be out-of-date and there will be treatments or even a cure. But as of this writing (2002), there truly aren't any.)

However, websites and books are out there usually because people want to make money. They want to convince you that there *is* a cure. You just haven't heard about it yet. It's a secret, it's new, and so not many people—perhaps not even your own doctor—know about it. Does this sound too good to be true? That's because it is.

I have been on the "other side" a bit in dealing with people who claim to have cures. That is because I have had them spam my site. ("Spam" is an unwanted advertisement usually posted through e-mail, mailing list, or on an Internet message board. It is a free, though usually very unwelcome and frowned upon, way of advertising.) Needless to say, I am not amused with spam. I offer my website for free as a support group for people with food allergies, and usually spend at least an hour a day with volunteer upkeep. It's not online for people to post advertisements in an effort to make money. When I wrote to one "doctor" who had spammed the FAST mailing list and told him that his way of advertising was inappropriate, he lashed out at me in an e-mail attacking me as a person (including my Christian religious beliefs) and claiming I wanted everyone with food allergies to be sick. This was a strange accusation, considering that I personally have severe food allergies. However, it helped convince me that I was right in taking a hard line against claims for cures. I personally will not believe there is a cure until I hear about it on the national news. Although I like and own "real" guinea pigs, I won't personally *become* a "guinea pig."

Some people would say I'm being cynical, but there is such a thing as healthy cynicism. This is what must be exercised when researching food allergies. Everything *cannot* be taken at face value. Just because something is in print does not mean it is necessarily true. On the Internet, anyone can set up a website about food allergies within minutes. I started my website when I was nineteen years old, after I got home from college one day. Within probably a very short time it was listed with major search engines and drawing in visitors. My own experience shows how easy it is for anyone—*anyone*—*to* set up a website about food allergies. This is why it's so important to take everything you read with a grain of salt...even if it's printed in a book that you find in the store—but especially if it's information found online.

That being said, Food Allergy Survivors Together is subject to being inaccurate. I am quick to admit that. It is "laypeople" which participate in the site rather than doctors or researchers. We are there not as a medical resource, but rather as an online support group. If you are in need of emotional support, recipes, and a place to "talk" to others who know what you're going through—and don't mind the occasional "grain of salt" that comes along with friendly discussion forums—please visit FAST at **http://www.angelfire.com/mi/FAST**. Make sure you remember to capitalize "FAST."

Also, be sure to ask your allergist for resources s/he recommends. This will hopefully help ensure that the information is trustworthy.

20

A Chapter for Those Who Don't Have Allergies

It may be that you're reading this book because a child, spouse, friend, or other loved one was recently diagnosed with food allergies. If that is the case, you likely feel overwhelmed and powerless to help him or her. Believe it or not, there are ways in which you *can* help. By reading this book, you have already shown that you care. You have taken a positive first step in finding out how your friend's condition will alter his or her life. Your mission can now be to make your friend (or family member) feel as "normal" as possible, but also to be supportive and understanding about his or her differences.

Perhaps this is the first chapter you turned to in the book. In case this is the situation, I would like to begin with some background information.

A lot of people think food allergies are merely a "trend diet," and, in fact, some people do use the excuse of having food allergies to support the trend diet they are on. I won't get into specifics, but there are books on the market that claim most people have food allergies, which is not true. Some people claim they are allergic to something just because they don't like it. However, in general, food allergies are quite real.

Your friend was probably born with food allergies, or at least a predisposition to develop them, probably in babyhood or early childhood. Symptoms of food allergies often first appear in babyhood when the child is first introduced to solid foods. If they are handled immediately (through avoidance of the problem food(s)), some children's allergies can regress and/or disappear. However, it has been assumed that most adults with food allergies will not be "cured," and allergies to certain foods are generally life-long.

Many people think I developed food allergies as a teen, which is when I was diagnosed. The truth is that I had them my entire life, but they progressively got worse. My reactions in childhood were so mild, or only came in spurts, that my parents and doctors thought they were unrelated. My symptoms as a child were things such as eczema, vomiting, stomachaches, and diarrhea. Perhaps your friend was also diagnosed later on in life. This doesn't mean that your friend just suddenly developed food allergies out of thin air. If you ask, your friend may be able to explain when s/he first noticed the symptoms.

Your friend probably was tested through either a skin-prick or blood test method by an allergist. This is sometimes followed by food challenging (if the allergy is not too severe) to determine that an allergy really is present. (Sometimes food allergies are discovered by a child's parents very early on. An example would be if a mom feeds her child peanut butter for the first time and the child can no longer breathe. A trip to the emergency room would probably verify that the child is allergic to peanuts. With this type of allergy, the last thing someone is going to want to do is to challenge the allergen! This is the most severe type of reaction, and is called "anaphylaxis.")

Food allergies are a serious condition. In the USA alone, around 100-200 people are reported to die every year from their food allergies. However, food allergies vary from person to person. Your friend may not have them as badly as someone else does, or may have them worse than others. If you ask, your friend would probably be happy to tell you how serious or mild his or her food allergies are.

Some people have such mild allergies that they really pose no imposition in their lives. Others' lives are severely impacted by their allergies. Food allergy reactions, however, should never be assumed to be "trivial." People with food allergies can have many symptoms, including acute stomach cramping, severe diarrhea, projectile vomiting, eczema, rashes, or even immediate death.

The terms "allergy" and "intolerance" are often erroneously used interchangeably. These are two different maladies, not to be confused with one another. Many of the times I hear from people who think they have a milk allergy, it may actually be lactose intolerance. Lactose intolerance is not related to food allergies; it is an entirely different problem and is not a disease, but instead the lack of an enzyme. If one's reaction to milk is very new and very mild (slight diarrhea, a stomachache or bloating), this is likely more indicative of lactose intolerance.

It is possible that you might not believe your friend about his or her reactions, and this is fully understandable. Many people with health problems tend to hide their symptoms to try to fit in, or because they don't want people to worry. When I have gotten really sick with my allergies I have been known to camp out in the bathroom (with the door locked) with a sleeping bag where no one can see me. Even when I have had public reactions (for example, I have vomited once, and fainted various times in school), no one seems to notice or attribute it to my food allergies. Surprisingly, people are very blasé about my reactions, even when I pass out.

Remember that your friend's reactions are possibly humiliating. It is never fun to be different, and your friend probably wants to appear as normal as possible. Because of this the reactions may be concealed. S/he may not even tell acquaintances that s/he has any health problems. When I had severe eczema behind my ears I always wore my hair down to hide it. Likewise, many people with food allergies will do all they can to hide their reactions.

Are you wondering how you can help? Here's a typical conversation between two people:

"Want to do something together?"

"Sure, let's go grab a bite to eat!"

Our culture is literally obsessed with food and eating out. Any time people want to "get together" with friends, family, or on a date, it's to eat—whether it's at a restaurant, potluck, or barbecue. Your friend may feel self-conscious about this. I personally stopped going to a church's youth meetings in part because the first 30 or so minutes of a 60-minute Sunday school class were devoted to eating! People with food allergies often feel alienated because so many outside activities involve food. Finding other activities to do with your friend who has food allergies will show that you care for your friend and don't just feel s/he is an excuse to have someone to eat with. (If you'd like, you can check out chapter seven for various activity ideas.)

It may be hard being friends with someone who can't do so-called "normal" things, but trust me—your friend appreciates you and your efforts. I think you will find that having a "special" friend is truly worth it!

Conclusion

Are you overwhelmed with information? If you read this book cover-to-cover, I am not surprised. Being diagnosed with food allergies—and the consequences that follow—can be overwhelming. It takes most of us years to get a handle on the disease. Even then, life has a way of throwing us for a loop. Your favorite prepackaged product may be discontinued, or one of your allergens may be added to it. You may lose a friend because s/he cannot handle being around someone who is "different."

It is my desire that this book will be there for you when something takes you by surprise. Keep it in a safe place. Remember there are others who have been through the same situations, the same difficulties, the same concerns. You are not alone.

APPENDIX

"My Tips for Someone Newly Diagnosed"

FAST members were asked to offer their personal tips for people who have recently been diagnosed with food allergies. Though the original question was for their number one tip, many couldn't think of just one!

Anna Patterson: "Try to include variety in your diet. For example, people seem to use soy in a lot of dishes, in addition to the soy that is already in many prepackaged foods. Variety is important so that you don't become bored with what you eat."

Nicole Melnick: "Don't take 'no' for an answer. If you feel that you are having an allergic reaction to foods—or anything for that matter—and you see a doctor who only runs the bare minimum of allergy tests, do not leave thinking you are not allergic to anything if the tests come back negative. It took several doctors to finally figure out all of my allergies. Get a second opinion. Get even a third or fourth."

Loretta Pearson: "It helps to know you're not alone and that there are others walking the food allergy trail. Finding another person with food allergies can be a great source of support and help."

Nicole Melnick: "Don't let anyone ever make you feel as if you are a problem or a burden. You are special in a good way! People may treat you as if your allergies are a burden on them, especially when it comes to social gatherings that revolve around food. My suggestion (and it works!): Offer to make something for a party or family gathering that you can eat (and know is allergen-free) that everyone else can partake in. You don't even have to tell anyone that it is allergen-free. Oftentimes, they won't even notice. And who knows…someone might even ask for the recipe."

Heather Cunningham: "Find a dietician—a good one who knows a lot about food allergies and stays up-to-date with current information—and make him or her a good friend. I have found that not all dieticians are equal, but we have one who has been more helpful to our family than any other one person."

Loretta Pearson: "For me a breakthrough came when I learned how to substitute new or different foods for the ones I can't eat. I learned to enjoy homemade salsa and other treats!"

Kim Pate: "I would say the best things I did when newly diagnosed included finding FAST (it has meant *so* much to know I'm not alone), allowing myself to 'splurge' on special foods, and learning how other cultures cook the things I can eat (so I greatly expand the ways I prepare my meals). It *can* be fun!"

Loretta Pearson: "Since I have a hard time eating in restaurants with so many food allergies, I've learned to make a few easy special foods that we use for our 'night out.' It's fun to know I made the delicious meal myself, and since it costs less to eat at home, we can have special foods we couldn't otherwise afford!"

Anna Patterson: "Read labels. Reread labels. Then check again. If the food is something you always eat, read the label whenever you buy it. Ingredients change."

Loretta Pearson: "I'm proud to be creating my own cookbook with recipes that are tailored just for my food allergies. There are great food allergy cookbooks out there, but if you have several allergies, then you still have to learn how to substitute for what you can't have in many of the recipes. So I'm making my own cookbook. It has 'my recipes' for my special food!"

Alysa Joaquin: "Never give up hope! Don't dwell on what you can't have, instead check out some recipe books from the library, look up some recipes on the Internet, and alter old recipes so that you can focus on what you *can* have. Look up substitutes too, so that if you can't have eggs you can still make cookies that call for eggs, only with an egg replacer. I've found it's also a good idea to put together your own cookbook, so you don't need to worry about sifting through foods you can't even think about having in an actual cookbook."

Mylène Belzile: "For traveling, I bought a plug-in hot pot (the kind you normally have for boiling water). This one is a small one where the top opens, and it is mentioned on the box that you can heat soup or water in it. I bring noodles, broth, and veggies along for the week (having access to a fridge—or even just a mini-bar—is a plus since you can bring perishables). I make myself soups, noodles with veggies, tomato sauce, spaghetti, and salads. I eat all three meals in my room. I normally try to get hotel rooms that have a kitchenette in them, since that is a lot better than making food from one little pot, but in case it is not possible, I have my little pot."

Kelsey McNitt: "First off, it's fine to be bewildered and scared, but don't panic. People can, and many *do*, live long, fairly normal lives with food allergies. Learn to read labels, call food companies, prepare your own foods, and be a little cautious, and go on living your life. Educating yourself and others should be a goal everyone with food allergies has. The more other people know about food allergies, the better they will understand the seriousness of them. They will also be able to understand that you aren't a furry green monster who can only eat pureed mush. People with food allergies are normal people who have jobs and families, go to school and daycare, play with friends, and have parties. Their bodies just react differently to certain foods, so their lifestyle is just a bit different from the 'average' person."

Loretta Pearson: "A good tip for eating in restaurants is to write down—*before* you go—the foods you want and how they need to be prepared. Example: 'I need a salad with *no* onions, cheese, eggs, or dressing.' By writing out what you need you won't forget to mention an important allergen. Also, if you need your food to be prepared in a special way, you might write something such as: 'Please sauté this in a clean pan, as cross-contamination is a serious threat to me.'"

Nicole Melnick: "Be your own investigator. There is a lot of information out there—some good (the FAST site), some bad. Many doctors are not all that familiar with allergies that do not cause immediate reactions and label people with delayed allergies as not being allergic, even though we react in the same manner as an allergic person (perhaps with just a delayed reaction). I have found some wonderful, helpful books and websites. However, I urge you to sift through all of the information you find and take everything you read with a grain of salt. There is a lot of misinformation out there."

Mylène Belzile: "After getting diagnosed with my allergies I noticed that by cooking all of my food myself I was seeing cooking in the same way I was seeing cleaning—as a daily chore I had to do, even if I didn't feel like it! I got to the point where I lost interest in food. Then, I thought to myself: 'Why not have a little fun and make myself a little treat? There's nothing stopping me if the foods are on my safe list.' So, once in a while when I get bored with my food I grab a few safe fruits (cookies are good, too), melt some safe chocolate, and eat chocolate-dipped fruits! I don't have to feel guilty about it (my diet is strict enough as it is). If I can find some safe chocolate, ice cream or donuts, there's nothing wrong with enjoying them when I feel like it."

About the Author

Melissa Taylor was medically diagnosed with food allergies as a teenager. In 1997 she started the website Food Allergy Survivors Together, located at **www.angelfire.com/mi/FAST** (remember to capitalize "FAST" if you visit). The website and its forums are intended to be a "virtual support group" for those who may not live near others with the same disorder. Recipes, cooking tips and emotional support are regularly exchanged on its forums.

Not to be defined by her health problems, Melissa enjoys playing with the family pets, reading, writing, drawing, making people laugh, doing impressions, and singing—much to the chagrin of others.

0-595-24128-X

Printed in the United States
R2046000001B/R20460PG43919LVSX00001B/1}